ALSO BY STEVEN PIRIANO

Josh and Joey's Incredible Museum Adventure

The Lost Ugew

MY STEPS FORWARD
AN INSPIRATIONAL GUIDE TO LIVING A BETTER LIFE

My Steps Forward
An Inspirational Guide to Living a Better Life

Steven Piriano

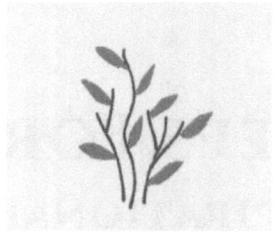

InspireGrowth

Copyright © 2021 by Steven Piriano

All rights reserved. No portion of this book may be reproduced in any manner without written permission from the publisher, except as permitted by United States copyright law.

For permissions, please contact:
InspireGrowth Enterprises
PO Box 119
Highland Mills, NY 10930

Book Design by ebooklaunch.com

Book Cover Design by ebooklaunch.com

For my family, my most beloved teachers

Contents

INTRODUCTION 1
CHAPTER 1: Standing Up to Bullies 5
CHAPTER 2: Career Confusion?
Do the Thing That Makes You Happy 9
CHAPTER 3: Finding Love 15
CHAPTER 4: CPR in Progress 21
CHAPTER 5: The Big C 25
CHAPTER 6: The Benefits of a Healthy Diet 33
CHAPTER 7: Lessons from a Penny 39
CHAPTER 8: Failure Equals Opportunity 47
CHAPTER 9: Expanding the Zone 57
CHAPTER 10: The Little Things 69
CHAPTER 11: Willpower? Not So Much 73
CHAPTER 12: Curveballs 77
CHAPTER 13: Perspectives 83
CHAPTER 14: Vantage Points 89
CHAPTER 15: Teachers 95
CHAPTER 16: A Backward Society? 105
CHAPTER 17: Clear Goals and Consistent Action 123
CHAPTER 18: You Are Unique 133
CHAPTER 19: Final Thoughts 137
AUTHOR'S NOTE 147
ENDNOTES 149

INTRODUCTION

Hello, and welcome!
   It is absolutely fantastic to have you here with me.
   Thank you for taking the time to read this book. I know how busy we can be, and the fact that you are here with me means a lot. In return for your time, it is my hope to give you some useful information that you can carry with you.
   I would like to begin by discussing my reasons for writing this book. I have been on this earth for fifty years. Thinking about that in cosmic terms, I have completed fifty trips around the sun. It sounds impressive when I phrase it like that, doesn't it? Throughout that time, I have come to appreciate the value of learning and growth. Looking back on my life thus far, a lot has happened. My time here has been filled with experiences and mentors who have provided a wealth of education and enabled me to grow emotionally, intellectually, and spiritually. Interestingly, many times this was happening even though I had no idea that I was being educated.
   Reflecting on my childhood, I did well in school and have enjoyed studying for as long as I can remember. Moreover, my desire for knowledge has grown. However, it wasn't until many years into adulthood that I began to have a thirst for understanding that would lead not only to greater book knowledge but also to my own

self-betterment. As it happens, a frightening health scare was the pivotal event that led my life down a different path. This new trajectory began with my desire to learn more about health. Over time, it unintentionally evolved into a yearning to improve all aspects of myself. I believe that my life experiences up to that point had left me receptive to what was about to happen.

I had my first exposure to personal development literature almost by coincidence. Although, I would like to share that I no longer believe in coincidences. As Albert Einstein once said, "Coincidence is God's way of remaining anonymous." In 2008, I was in a grocery store when I happened to pass by the magazine aisle. I always like to browse the titles, and there was one in particular that caught my eye. It was there that I picked up my first issue of a well-known personal development publication.

I consumed it over the next few days and felt empowered by what it had taught me. This then led me to purchase a book that had been featured in that magazine, and I was thrilled by the things that it illuminated for me. This led to the purchase of another book by a different author. I developed insights that I had never had before, which resulted in the purchase of yet another book, and then another book, and so on. My appetite for knowledge and ideas to help me improve as a person continues to grow.

I want to be the best person I can be. I have gifts and talents I want to cultivate and share with others. Moreover, I am not unique in this. *Every single one of us* has gifts and talents. We all have something special to offer the world. Furthermore, this contribution to humankind does not have to be something grandiose and earth-changing to be significant. I believe that every action you perform and every word you utter has the potential to add value to others. A few things that can have a great positive influence on others come to mind: coaching a children's soccer team, giving piano lessons, planting a vegetable garden, holding the door for the person behind you, and raising your children with love.

I would like to tell you some of the stories from my life that helped shape me. I have learned countless valuable lessons through the experiences I've had, as well as from other people (many times from family and friends and many times via their thoughts, written down in the books I've read). Each of these helped me to improve in some way. Looking back, I can see that they all encouraged me to take small steps forward on the path of my life. It is these anecdotes and lessons that I would like to share with you. It is my hope that they may teach you something, perhaps help you to see things a bit differently, and maybe even help you to improve your life in some way.

CHAPTER 1

STANDING UP TO BULLIES

In relating stories from my life, I'd like to begin by briefly mentioning my earlier years. I was born in Brooklyn, New York, and I have twin sisters that arrived four years later. My parents divorced when I was around ten years old, and we moved back and forth a few times between Brooklyn and Staten Island. There were also times when we had no home, and stayed with family, friends or in motels. Although there were many difficult periods growing up, there were certainly good times as well. I hold memories of picnics, swimming pools, Cub Scouts, birthday parties and Christmas mornings.

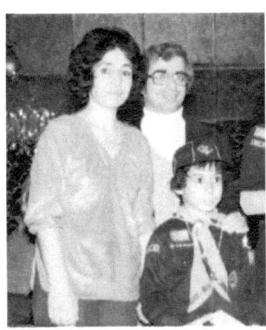 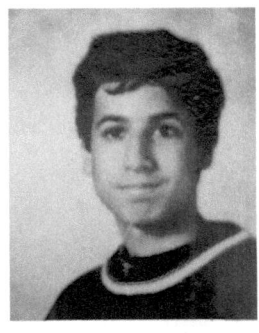

Me as a Cub Scout with my parents.   Me in junior high school

Junior high school found me back in Brooklyn. As a kid of this age, I was skinny and really smart. Sounds like a pretty good combination of traits to have, doesn't it? Well, it turns out that in junior high, it increases the likelihood of being bullied. And yes, I was one of the lucky ones who got bullied. I was picked on both verbally and physically. I was called names and made fun of on a fairly consistent basis. I can remember one time when we were playing Wiffle ball during gym period. I was wearing sweatpants, and every time I was up at bat, the catcher of the opposing team would yank them down. Although I told him to stop multiple times, my efforts seemed to be in vain. I think that I was not speaking from a place of strength and conviction. In addition, for whatever reason, my gym teacher did not see this horrible act that was taking place. That was, by far, the most humiliating game of Wiffle ball that I ever played. Thankfully, I did have a small group of friends. Moreover, sometimes one of the bigger kids in my group stood up for me. But because I was not always with them, my little circle of friends did not offer consistent protection.

The memories of being bullied that remain the clearest in my mind are those times after eighth period. Eighth period was the last period of the day, and for me it was Italian class. After this last period, everyone would walk back to their homerooms to get ready for dismissal from school for the day. I'm not sure how this began, but there was a group of three kids from my Italian class who would follow me back to my homeroom and take turns slapping the back of my neck the entire way. It was hurtful and embarrassing. This occurred *every single day.* I knew that other people saw what was happening, and this only made it worse. I absolutely dreaded eighth period because I knew what was coming right after the bell rang.

The girl who sat next to me during Italian class also knew what was happening. I clearly remember her saying that I should not let them hit me. She told me that I should stand up for myself. She told me this many times. I really wanted to take her advice, but I was afraid. *What if I did something and they hit me even harder? What if they actually beat me up right there in the middle of a hallway packed with other kids? What then? What would I do? What could I do?*

Consequently, this neck-slapping ritual of theirs went on for a while longer. Then the day finally arrived. I was not planning for it to happen that day, but it did. It was a typical day. Eighth period Italian. The bell rang and the class ended. Next came the walk back to homeroom and both the literal pain in the neck I was about to experience and the further striking down of my self-esteem. My hallway buddies did not disappoint. *Slap. Slap. Slap.* I felt as if I was about to cry. Yes, right there in the middle of the hallway, I felt tears stinging the backs of my eyes. It was at that point that I had had enough. Something happened inside me, and it took only a few seconds to put my fear aside. I turned around and slapped one of my aggressors really hard on the back of *his* neck. My heart was pounding, and I was breathing fast. I immediately ran back to my homeroom. I was scared, but I felt good. I had stood up for myself. That was the last day those kids bullied me.

Takeaways

- Sometimes it takes becoming truly fed up and disgusted with something to enact a change.
- It takes only a few seconds of courage to do something that can be life-altering.
- Stand up for yourself in situations where you are being oppressed. *Important caveat: Except in true self-defense situations, violence is not a good solution.* I did hit another kid. But it left no mark and did no real harm. Well-chosen words are a far better way to show strength than using your fists.

CHAPTER 2

CAREER CONFUSION? DO THE THING THAT MAKES YOU HAPPY

Moving forward a few years, past junior high school and into high school, I was significantly better off in the bullying department. There were still several bullies roaming about, but I was never seriously picked on. By this time, I had a slightly larger circle of close friends whom I was often with. I was still smart and enjoyed studying, but I was not made to feel small because of it. Biology became one of my favorite subjects, which I suppose was a foreshadowing for the academic and, subsequently, career expedition that I would eventually embark on.

As for the professional paths that I explored, two people had a great influence on me. One of them was my dad. He was a locksmith at a large public hospital in Brooklyn. Along with the children's books about the human body that he gave me, he also brought me a few trinkets that he had come across. By trinkets, I mean plastic models of the human heart and brain.

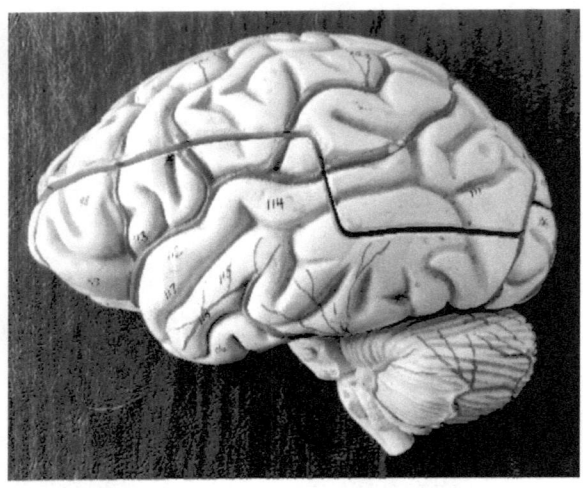

My Plastic Brain Model

I was amazed by these objects and by the things that I learned from the books. It was at that time that I believe my journey toward becoming a physician began. My grandpa Nick was the other individual who had an influence on my eventual choice of educational venues. He had a great interest in fiddling with electrical appliances and electronics. He knew a lot and could always fix things when they broke. He taught me about resistors, transistors, and capacitors. He showed me how to use a voltmeter and read schematic diagrams. If he were alive today, I'm sure that he would be amazed at the way the field of technology has exploded. Anyway, I ended up taking an electronics class in high school that furthered my interest in the subject.

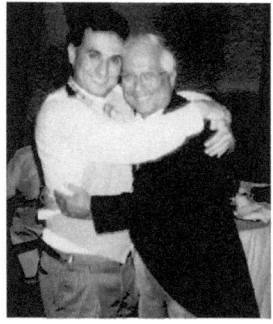
Me and my dad

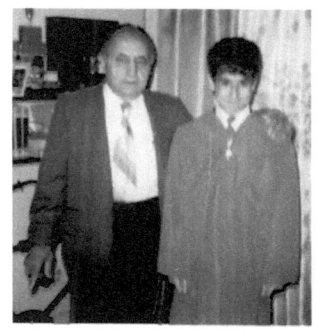
Me and my Grandpa Nick

When junior year rolled around, it was time to decide which college to attend and what I wanted to do for the rest of my life. Thinking about the subjects of the human body and electronics, I had a greater interest in the former. I was in awe of the way everything in the human body worked so perfectly together. I also wanted to do something to help people. All things considered, it seemed as though becoming a doctor was the obvious answer to the question of which career path I should follow.

However, there was one small problem. Commitment. Over the years, I had heard that becoming a doctor required a huge sacrifice. People told me that to pursue this career, medicine would overwhelm every other area of my life. This frightened me. I was not sure if I wanted to pledge loyalty to something that would take up so much of my time. I was confused for several months. After much deliberation, I finally decided that the commitment was not worth it. At this point, I decided to enter the field of electrical engineering, based on my interest in electronics.

I applied to several colleges and ended up enrolling at Polytechnic University in Farmingdale, New York. My course load included chemistry, calculus, computer science, and physics. I really enjoyed physics. However, I could not say the same for the other classes, especially computer science and calculus. I just could not wrap my brain around many of the concepts. I ended up getting a D in Calculus I. I took it over and got an A. I repeated this cycle with both Calculus II and III. As far as I can recall, I don't believe that I did so great in computer science either. The subjects that were the foundation for engineering were turning out not to be as I had envisioned them. I started to question my decision to become an electrical engineer.

To say that it was a time of confusion is an understatement. There I was, having completed nearly two years of undergraduate studies, and I was clueless about what I wanted to be when I grew up. I spoke with counselors at the college and took computer-based personality inventories to see what careers might be a good fit for me. The results of these assessments all pointed to one thing—becoming a physician. I thus found myself back at square one. I was quite sure that the commitment required to be a physician had not gotten any easier, and this still scared me.

There are certain moments in life that you will remember forever. They will always remain with you, not because of their emotional content but because they were pivotal; they somehow altered the course of your life. One such moment for me occurred one night after I returned home from work. I worked part-time throughout my senior year of high school, as well as during the summers while in college, as a waiter at a Sizzler restaurant. It was late in the evening, and I remember sitting in the living room with my dad. I told him how confused I was. Everything seemed to be pointing to me becoming a doctor, but I was afraid. I don't remember his exact words, but I'll paraphrase. He said, "You have to do something that you like. You don't want to go to work every day and be miserable with what you are doing. If you can see yourself doing and enjoying what a doctor does, then that is what you should do. Don't worry so much about the commitment. If you're happy being a doctor, then you'll be happy to make the commitment."

That conversation changed the course of my life. It was at that moment that I decided to go for it. It was a lot of work. I applied to other colleges while I was still attending Polytechnic. Eventually, I was accepted to the premed program at Brooklyn College. I learned a lot and had a great time. I also enjoyed working as a peer tutor in biology while there. Because some of my credits from Polytechnic did not transfer, I spent three years at Brooklyn College, for a total of five years as an undergraduate.

During the latter part of my undergraduate experience, I began the medical school application process. I took the MCAT (Medical College Admission Test) and did well. I applied to several schools and received a rejection letter from each one. I thus decided to continue my studies at Brooklyn College as a nonmatriculated graduate student and to become certified as an EMT. I did this for a year and then reapplied to medical school.

It wasn't too long before the eagerly awaited letter finally arrived in the mail. All I wanted to see was the first line. Was it going to contain the all-too-familiar "We regret to inform you ... ," or would it say something to the effect of "Congratulations"? I slowly opened the envelope and unfolded the paper inside. My eyes gradually moved down the letter until they came upon the words that indicated my acceptance into medical school. I was overjoyed. I was also alone. My dad was out of town on vacation. I had nobody to share my news with. I did manage to track him down through his hotel concierge (no cell phones back then) and shared the great news. He was ecstatic. And so began my journey into the field of medicine.

Takeaways

- You should always do what makes you happy. Put another way, if you are drawn to a project or career, you should not eschew it solely because of fear. That might lead to regret and always asking yourself "What if?"

- Other people often see life from different perspectives, which can many times help make difficult choices a bit easier.

- Commitment is not all that bad. As a matter of fact, commitment is a necessity for any worthwhile undertaking. Moreover, if you are enjoying the work you are doing, the commitment you make becomes a gratifying and pleasurable experience.

CHAPTER 3

FINDING LOVE

Medical school was quite an experience. It required an enormous amount of dedication and work. I attended medical school in Brooklyn from 1994 to 1998. The first two years consisted of the basic science courses, including gross anatomy, pathophysiology, biochemistry, pathology, microbiology, and pharmacology. The last two years comprised clinical clerkships and electives. It was during these years that we worked in doctors' offices and hospitals and participated in real patient care.

There were many late nights of studying, especially during the first two years. My two closest friends and I would find a table and chairs in an isolated corner of a hallway and spend time either there or in an empty classroom, studying into the early-morning hours. I'll always remember one particular night when we were studying hard for an exam. It must have been one o'clock in the morning, and we were getting hungry. We took a taxi to a burger place in Manhattan that we liked. We sat and ate with our neuroscience notes spread out and covering the entire table. Ah, the memories.

It wasn't all work, though. There was playtime interspersed between the schoolwork. I had a close-knit group of friends, and we went out regularly and had a good time. I have fond memories of being with my friends in restaurants, dance clubs, and other get-togethers. You know what they say about all work and no play. It was these enjoyable times outside of studying that helped give my brain a necessary rest.

After three years of hardcore studying, the fourth and final year had arrived at last. At this time, I found myself facing another dilemma. It was during the fourth year that we were supposed to decide which field of medicine, and thus what type of residency training program, we wanted to pursue. We had been exposed to many different medical specialties during the prior year, and decision time had arrived. I was in a quandary. I enjoyed both anesthesiology and emergency medicine and could not decide between the two. After spending additional elective time in each discipline and speaking with my mentor in the emergency department at Kings County Hospital in Brooklyn, I finally decided on emergency medicine.

I matched into a training program that started with a year of internal medicine followed by three years of emergency medicine. It was an exciting time of education and growth, during which I learned the art and science of emergency medicine. It was also a time of love. During my intern year, we were paired up with third-year medical students who were doing their clinical clerkships. An exceptionally beautiful young woman was assigned to be with me. However, because I was so focused on the work that needed to be done for the day, I was oblivious to the great treasure who stood before me. I politely introduced myself and shook her hand. Then I left and proceeded to ignore her. I later found out that she was pretty upset about that.

Over the next week or so, I started behaving the way I should have from the very beginning. I spoke with this young woman and taught her whatever I could about the patients we cared for. I became drawn to her. We had daily noon lectures, during which lunch was served (sandwiches every day). It was sometimes difficult to pay attention to the speaker because I was admiring my student from across the room. I thought (and hoped) that the feeling was mutual. I finally decided to find out and came up with a plan—and the courage—to ask her out.

I wanted to wait until her clerkship was over. It was the Wednesday before Thanksgiving break. While all the other students were sent home early, I asked my student if she wanted to stay a bit later and practice starting an IV on me. I later found out that she was not too happy about being asked to remain behind when most of her friends had already been dismissed. After practicing IVs on me (and my sore forearm), we both went back to our call room. This is where I had planned to ask for a date. There was small talk for a few minutes, and then, when I finally mustered up enough bravery to ask this especially important question, someone walked into the room and started talking to us. Finally ... the person left. More small talk followed, and I worked myself back up to the question. Then someone else walked in and struck up a conversation. Really? This happened about three or four times. I was eventually granted a few minutes alone with her and, with my heart racing, managed to get the words out of my mouth.

Her response hit me kind of hard. She said that she needed to study and didn't have time to go out. I was quite disappointed. I mentally picked myself back up and moved on to plan B. I gave her my phone number and told her that if she ever wanted to take a study break, she could give me a call. A few days later, the eagerly awaited call came. We had a wonderful first date—dinner and a movie. While enjoying our first meal together, she would eat the crust of the bread and discard the fluffy white inside, which was my favorite part. At that point, I knew we were meant for each other.

Although our clinical rotation had ended, we spent a lot of time together and grew closer. A few years later, after much careful planning, we were out on a picnic at Clove Lakes Park in Staten Island, New York. There were grapes, cheese, and lots of little clues written on sticky notes. It was there that I got down on one knee, holding a ring in my hand, and asked that stunning young woman to marry me. To my great pleasure, she said yes, and we've been inseparable ever since.

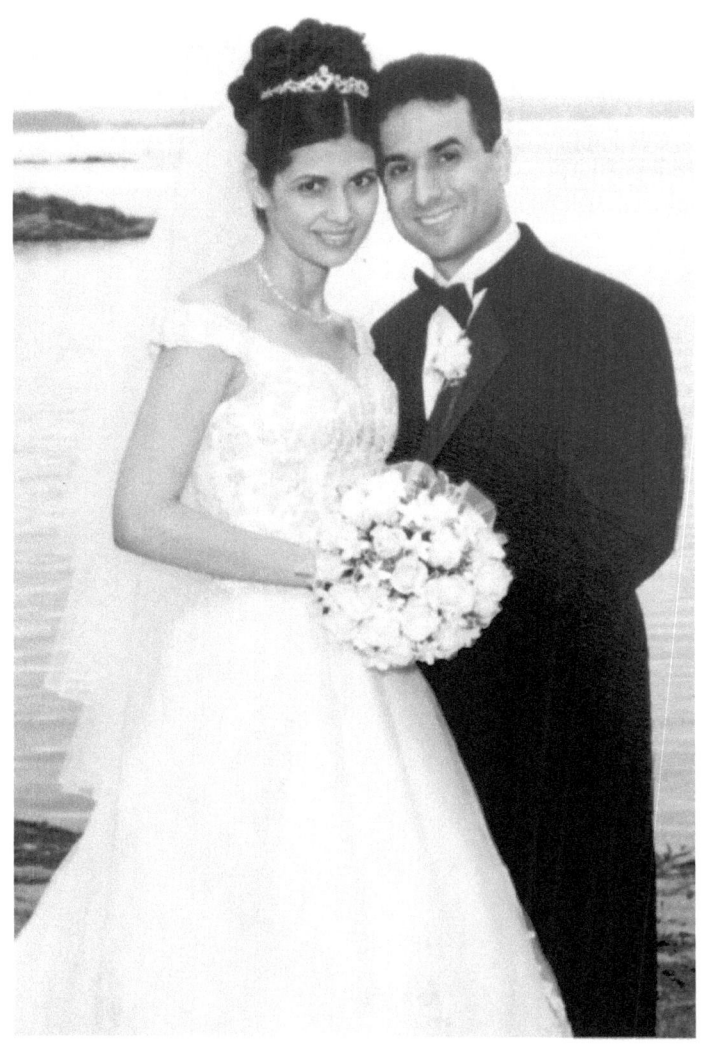

Me and my beautiful bride

Takeaways

- Allowing your brain time for rest and relaxation will enhance both your creativity and productivity.
- Love is powerful and can enable one to discover courage.

CHAPTER 4

CPR IN PROGRESS

Following residency training, I became a full-fledged emergency medicine physician. I worked hard and continued learning. My ongoing education came in the form of book learning and, more importantly, experiential learning. I was caring for patients with all sorts of maladies—everything from pneumonia, asthma, and bronchitis to severe flare-ups of emphysema. I treated everything from broken fingers and toes to patients who were victims of major traumas, such as car accidents, falls out of windows, stabbings, and gunshot wounds. I was tasked with differentiating benign rashes from those that heralded a life-threatening systemic illness. In addition, over the years, I have taken care of countless people suffering from diabetes, high blood pressure, heart disease, stroke, and cancer. I learned how to manage exacerbations of these chronic medical conditions with lifesaving medications. It is an incredibly rewarding experience to see people who were once in extreme physical distress resting more comfortably because of the treatments that I rendered.

During the course of my early career, I practiced medicine and saved many lives. However, at some point, I started to notice a trend that I had not previously appreciated. It seemed that people were being stricken at younger ages by what I had formerly believed were "old people diseases." There are patients scattered throughout the years whom I remember quite well. One such patient arrived on a sunny afternoon in the middle of a typical busy shift.

We received the call from EMS. It was a cardiac arrest with CPR in progress. Several minutes later, the patient was rushed in through the ambulance bay doors. A paramedic was at her side doing chest compressions as she was wheeled into our resuscitation room. I was immediately struck by how young this woman looked. I was informed that she was thirty-nine years old. I remember thinking, *Thirty-nine years old? What's going on? This can't be a typical heart attack. Thirty-nine-year-olds don't have heart attacks.* We worked on her for a long time. We continued CPR and gave her multiple rounds of medications to try to restart her heart. No response. A glance at the monitor during a pulse check showed a flatline. More CPR and additional medications were administered. I did not want to give up. I did not want to lose this young woman, who probably had a family. More CPR. More medications. Still a flatline. Although I didn't want to stop, it seemed that I had to accept the fact that further efforts would be futile. With a heavy heart, I called an end to the resuscitation efforts and pronounced a time of death. I still could not understand. *How could this happen? There had to be something else going on.*

The patient ended up being a medical examiner's case, and an autopsy was performed. To my great dismay, the cause of death was determined to be a coronary artery occlusion. This unfortunate young woman did indeed have her life taken by a heart attack. Prior to that time, I had never heard of a heart attack occurring in someone so young.

My initial shock slowly disappeared, and life in the emergency department continued. As the months wore on, though, I began to take notice of an increasing number of younger individuals seeking care for conditions such as diabetes, cancer, heart disease, and strokes. I took care of them to the best of my ability. But I still wondered, *What was going on?* Much more on this to come.

Takeaways

- Education via experience adds an entirely new depth of knowledge to book learning.
- The fact that young people are getting "old people diseases" should prompt the question "Why?"

CHAPTER 5

THE BIG C

I will always remember September 7, 2007. That Friday brought us a bright and mild morning, and I was off from work. We were getting ready to take our two boys, at that time approaching their third and first birthdays, to the park. I was looking forward to a great time outdoors, until one event drastically changed the trajectory of both my day and my life.

After I got ready, I used the bathroom to urinate and ended up doing a double take. The toilet water was crimson. For a moment, I thought I was dreaming. But after staring into the toilet for a minute, I knew that I was indeed experiencing reality. I had just urinated blood. I was confused for a short time. *What could this mean?* As a physician, I had several ideas of what this symptom could indicate, and I knew I had to get it checked out.

I told my wife what had happened, and I made some phone calls. Instead of heading out to the park, we drove over to a urologist's office. He thought that it might be a kidney stone. But that assessment sounded strange, because I knew that kidney stones were often painful, and I had no pain. However, he wanted to be sure and evaluate this possibility further, so he ordered a CAT scan. I walked across the street to the hospital where I worked and in a short time found myself lying down in the CAT scan machine.

I knew everyone who worked in the department, and I was also quite familiar with the CAT scan process. The stretcher glides into the machine, and images are acquired over about a minute, after which the technician comes back into the room and helps the patient off the table. After I lay down, my body moved into and back out of the machine. The scan was done. I waited for the technician to reenter the room. *It's taking a really long time for her to come back,* I thought. *Too long.* I stared at the ceiling and back at the door. *Something isn't right.*

The door finally opened. But it was not the technician who walked into the room. It was one of the radiologists. I thought, *OK, something is definitely wrong.* The radiologist, who I knew well, looked me in the eyes and, in a concerning yet matter-of-fact tone, said, "Steve, you have a mass on your right kidney." *A mass?* They helped me off the table and into the control room. I studied the images of my internal organs on the monitor. There was indeed a grapefruit-size mass on my right kidney. I started to get a bit shaky but told myself that I needed to stay calm. *Is this really happening?*

I walked back to the car, where my wife and two sons were waiting. "I have a mass on my right kidney." My wife stared at me for a moment with a worried expression. My children, of course, were too young to understand the implications. We walked back into the urologist's office, and he studied the images on his monitor as well.

"It definitely looks like cancer," he said. "We need to take the kidney out."

"The whole kidney?" I asked.

"Yes," he replied. "The mass is too large. The kidney has to be removed."

I had known this doctor for a few years, and I had great trust in him. This made the process so much easier. The surgery was planned for a Monday evening. Things were moving fast. It almost seemed surreal, in a way. My weekend changed from a nice day in the park to the scheduled removal of my right kidney in the not-too-distant future.

After we returned home later that afternoon, there were several phone calls to be made. I telephoned each of my parents. My mother lived about two hours away in Brooklyn, and my father lived in Florida. They would both end up coming to my home and staying with me awhile.

I'll always remember the phone conversation with my dad. I could hear the extreme despondency in his voice. "I'm coming up," he said, his voice cracking. Although my dad and I are very close, those words nevertheless touched me deeply. He flew in the next day. (Later on, he told us he was so nervous he had somehow managed to board the wrong plane and only found out when the flight attendant announced the flight's destination before takeoff. Luckily, he managed to get off and still catch his flight.)

Our house was filled with people the next day. It was a show of love and concern, and I greatly appreciated it. That weekend also found me scheduled for a test called a bone scan. It was part of a process called staging, during which possible spread of a cancer, also called metastasis, is evaluated. Because renal cancer can often spread to bone, I was getting a scan of my bones. *No problem. I'm sure the cancer is isolated to my kidney,* I remember thinking at the time. *The bone scan will be normal; I'll have the surgery and be done with it.* I certainly maintained a positive outlook.

Things did not go exactly as planned. I remember looking at the bone scan with another one of my radiology colleagues. She called me into the radiology reading room with a concerned look on her face. *Oh no, not again.* She gestured to her monitor, which displayed an image of my skeleton. Everything looked normal. Everything except those two black circles in my left thigh bone. This meant that the cancer might have already spread. At this point, I began to worry. My positive outlook transformed into one of fear.

That night, I cried with my wife. *Is this really going to be the end for me? Am I not going to be able to grow old with my wife? Am I not going to be able to watch my two little boys grow up?* I knelt by my sons' bedsides, praying and crying. I asked God, if it was in His plans, if I might be able to spend more time with my family.

The next step was to get an MRI of my femur, to see if those black circles noted on the bone scan were cancerous. After the test, I sat in the corridor with my wife and brother-in-law, anxiously awaiting the results. It wasn't long before my radiology colleague, the same gentleman who had informed me of the kidney mass, reported to me that the lesions in my femur were benign. They were unrelated to the malignancy. It was as though a great weight had been lifted from my shoulders. I thanked God for giving me a chance.

The day of surgery was a bit unpleasant. My procedure was scheduled for the evening, and I had to be prepared for it. I was NPO (or *nil per os*)—nothing by mouth. In other words, I was starving. To make matters worse, I not only had to be empty from above but also from below. That was accomplished by an enema, which I enjoyed even less than being NPO. After registering at the hospital and waiting a bit, my wife and father were hungry. I laugh at it now, but at the time I was not too enthusiastic about sitting with them in the cafeteria while my own stomach growled.

The surgery went well that evening. My surgeon and colleague said that he got the kidney and the entire tumor. I spent a few days in the hospital hooked up to a morphine pump, with a tube in my nose. Although I can still recall the pain and nausea, something else stands out in my mind much more clearly—people. My room was often filled with people. I was visited by family, friends, and colleagues. They brought food and flowers. I was amazed by and so appreciative of all those who visited me. The amount of love and caring that I felt truly was a healing experience.

I was blessed for having so many people supporting me. I was even more blessed for having that one person who never left my side. My wife was there, in my room, 24-7. She slept in a recliner beside my hospital bed. If I got up at night, she got up at night. When I was in pain, she called for a nurse. When it was time for me to walk to the nursing station, she was right there, holding my hand. She gave me 110 percent of herself.

The trust and admiration I had for my surgeon was also therapeutic. During his daily visits, he was friendly, funny, and reassuring. He cracked jokes and maintained an emotional connection with both my wife and me. He put his hand on my shoulder. He made sure I was involved in my own recovery. I will always be thankful for him.

I was discharged from the hospital that Friday and went home to recover. I was enrolled in a clinical trial, which meant that I was soon going to start taking oral chemotherapy for a year. I took a medical leave of absence from work. I was about to have an extended rest, and, although I did not realize it at the time, my eyes were about to be opened to an entire world of knowledge that I had previously been blind to.

Life can change in an instant. My vision had been that I was going to grow old with my wife and raise my boys. That perspective was threatened for a time, and I realized that I had been taking many things for granted. This taught me to appreciate the wonderful things that I have in my life—treasures such as my wife's smile, my sons' laughter, and the fact that I can see, hear, walk, and talk. Admittedly, I am a fallible human and don't always show gratitude. But I strive to be better every day, and I'm happy about that. After all, I am blessed enough to be alive and well in 2021, and I do give thanks for that every day.

Besides coming to realize the importance of gratitude, I discovered that companionship and love can facilitate healing. My circle of friends and family taught me this. However, the most influential teacher of this lesson was my wife, Mayra. She was there all the time, never leaving my side. I don't think I had ever witnessed such selfless behavior before that, and I am grateful and humbled that some of it rubbed off on me.

Takeaways

- Appreciate and be thankful for the good things in your life.
- Friendship and connectedness can heal the body and the soul.

CHAPTER 6

THE BENEFITS OF A HEALTHY DIET

Not long after my hospital discharge, Mayra and I ventured into a Barnes & Noble bookstore in Manhattan. I entered the store with a few questions. *Why did I get cancer? I mean, I thought I had been eating healthy. Can my diet be improved? Should I exercise more? Is there anything else I should be doing to try to prevent this from happening again?* My goal was to purchase some books that could help me answer these queries. I found a few books on the subjects of cancer, as well as nutrition and healing, and a gentle excitement surged through me. I could not wait to get home to crack one of them open and begin what would become a new adventure.

As I dove into my first book, I started out intrigued. However, in a short time, I found myself fascinated by the information I was absorbing. I was also astonished to learn that the healthy lifestyle I thought I had been living all the years prior was, in fact, not so healthy after all.

Up to that time, I had been eating a lot of cereals, sandwiches, cheeses, granola bars, and instant meals that came in a bag. Therefore, the prevailing theme of my diet was primarily processed foods. Although I was not eating many cakes and other sweets, I was still eating plenty of foods that came in a bag or a box. Even as a trained physician, I was oblivious to the fact that I was eating poorly. The other major problem with my diet was that it was seriously lacking in the fruits and vegetables department. To be fair, I did consume fruits and vegetables on occasion, but they were not on the menu every day.

In all honesty, I had no idea that processed foods were at all unhealthy. I can still recall one evening when I was a young boy, maybe ten years old. My sisters and I were having our usual after-dinner dessert: cake. I had learned of a condition called diabetes, and I asked my mother if eating too much cake could lead to diabetes. She responded, "No, don't be silly." It wasn't until many years afterward that I learned that her response was not totally accurate. Of course, she was not intentionally trying to mislead me, but a lot of the knowledge regarding healthier diets was not discovered until decades later. Moreover, cakes and other sweets are not alone in the category of processed foods. Many cereals, breads, pastas, baked goods, and instant meals also fall into this classification.

Why are processed foods harmful? Many books have been written on the subject by people more qualified than me to discuss this topic. Nonetheless, I would like to provide a brief summary of changes that occur in our bodies when we consume processed foods regularly. The following is by no means a comprehensive description. However, I believe that it provides some key highlights.

One of the principal dangers of these foods is the rate at which they are broken down by the body. First, it is important to become aware of a scale known as the glycemic index. In simple terms, it provides a measurement of the speed with which a specific food will be broken down and release its carbohydrates (sugars) into the bloodstream. In general, processed foods have a higher glycemic index, which means that, after eating these foods, there will be a rapid rise in blood sugar. (Note, however, that there are some cereals, breads, and pastas that do have a lower glycemic index.) The body responds by doing what it is supposed to do to accommodate an increase in blood sugar—the cells of the pancreas release the hormone insulin. Because the blood sugar increases rapidly, there will be a large spike in insulin.

Over time, with the regular consumption of processed foods several times a day, the body's tissues and organs are constantly seeing high levels of insulin. Consequently, over time, these tissues and organs become less sensitive to the body's own insulin. The body will compensate by producing more and more of the hormone. If nothing changes, this decreased sensitivity eventually leads to insulin resistance.

It is at this point that things really go bad. Insulin resistance brings with it a whole host of disorders. When the body is in the throes of insulin resistance, it will develop fat accumulation around the waist, otherwise known as central obesity. This will be accompanied by high blood pressure and high triglycerides. Eventually, the cells of the pancreas will wear out and be unable to produce insulin. As a result, diabetes will become imminent. Some may feel that diabetes is perhaps not so bad. For those individuals, it is critical to understand that diabetes greatly increases the risks of developing heart attacks, strokes, kidney disease, vascular disease, and extremity gangrene, with the eventual need for limb amputations.

The most unfortunate thing, to me anyway, is that many of these horrendous medical conditions are likely preventable. I care for people who suffer from these conditions every day I go to work. I don't just read about these diseases in newspapers and magazines. I speak with and touch the countless people who are afflicted with these illnesses. I see firsthand how it affects both my patients and their families. One of the hardest parts of my job is notifying a family member that their loved one has just died. It is a conversation that I dread having as much today as I did when I first began practicing emergency medicine. My young, thirty-nine-year-old female patient who succumbed to a heart attack was the first in a very long list of people whose deaths may have been prevented.

My purpose in telling these stories is not to instill fear. What I would really like to do is create awareness and inspire action. My goal is to generate a desire in you, the reader, to become healthier. That is my aspiration. I would like people to know that they have many choices when it comes to eating healthier and feeling energetic and fantastic. To this end, I would like to spend a little time discussing fruits and vegetables.

Regarding the glycemic index, most fruits and vegetables are low on the scale. This signifies that their carbohydrates are released more slowly into the body. As a result, insulin is released more slowly, and the insulin spikes that occur after the consumption of processed foods are not seen. Thus, if a person's diet consists of an abundance of fruits and vegetables and lesser portions of processed foods, the metabolic path leading to eventual insulin resistance is less likely to be taken. Hence, the risk of developing obesity, high blood pressure, diabetes, and many other debilitating diseases becomes significantly lower.

Aside from the low glycemic index of most fruits and vegetables, another salient consideration is that they are packed with nutrients that the body needs—valuable vitamins, minerals, and antioxidants can be found in these foods. Furthermore, these substances are essential in helping to maintain good health and in lowering the risk of developing many of the diseases mentioned earlier as well as many types of cancer.

Personally, I enjoy eating nutritious foods, not only because of the health benefits but also because I genuinely like them. I feel clear, clean, and energetic after I eat them. In addition, they are versatile—they can be mouthwatering in recipes, and many are delicious when eaten by themselves.

The months following my cancer diagnosis were enlightening ones. I was provided with an opportunity to become aware of one of the most basic things in my life—the foods I was eating. Prior to this time, I thought that my diet was healthy overall. How mistaken I was. Although being diagnosed with cancer was terrifying, I am genuinely happy to have had the experience. It was the impetus that led to the process of self-education and a critical change in my lifestyle. Frequently, individuals or situations show up for a reason. They have come to impart a lesson. Moreover, to assimilate the ideas that are being offered, we must be receptive to them, even if it frightens us. In 2007, kidney cancer was my teacher, and I've had many more since then.

Takeaways

- Be open-minded. Often, people or circumstances enter our lives for a purpose. They have come to teach us something. What teachers have you had in your life?
- Eat a healthy diet. Consume an abundance of fruits and vegetables and a lesser amount of processed foods.

CHAPTER 7

LESSONS FROM A PENNY

Regarding diet, I do feel that learning about the types of foods one eats is important, as evidenced by the eye-opening knowledge I wrote about in the previous chapter, which was the spark that ignited my own change in eating habits. However, I do still try to keep it simple. The majority of the time, I eat foods that are as close to nature as possible. Fruits, vegetables, whole grains, beans, nuts, and seeds have become staples of my diet. Some of the foods I love are whole-grain rolled oats, blueberries, almond-milk yogurt, hummus, cashews, almonds, quinoa, grapes, bananas, apples, beans, flax and chia seeds, broccoli, and peppers.

I eat these types of foods most of the time. Concerning eating habits, and anything for that matter, *consistency is key*. If a person wants to eat healthy, it is what they do most of the time that counts. Eating one salad is not going to make you healthy, just as eating one cheeseburger is not going to give you a heart attack. However, eating a salad every day will make you healthier, just as eating a cheeseburger daily will likely affect your health in a negative manner. It is what you do most of the time, every day, over the course of months, that will begin to have an influence. I do love healthy foods. But every so often I will also enjoy a cookie or other sweet treat. I believe that this is OK because I am consistent in providing my body with wholesome foods most of the time.

Consistency and choices. I don't know the exact number of choices the average person makes on a daily basis. Nonetheless, I am sure that it is quite a large amount. Everything we do is a choice. From what we decide to eat to how we spend our days—these are all choices. Furthermore, over time, the choices a person makes will have an enormous effect on their life. It is vital to appreciate the fact that, aside from drastic decisions, the seemingly simple choices that a person makes every day will typically take a long time to manifest visible results in one's life; these results, though obvious, will occur gradually over time. It is also important to remember that these outcomes can be positive or negative.

Eat poorly most of the time and you will likely feel OK. You may notice that you are gaining weight and maybe feel a bit fatigued. After several years, your doctor may inform you that you are a diabetic and have high blood pressure. Continue making similar choices and you may end up in the emergency department with a heart attack. Conversely, eat healthy foods most of the time and you will notice a progressively greater feeling of well-being, higher energy levels, and increased focus. You will reap the rewards of your consistently good lifestyle choices.

To demonstrate the immense power of consistent small changes occurring slowly over time, I would like to tell the story of a penny. Not just any penny, but a very special penny. I'm sure that many have heard about what has been called the magic penny. You know it—take a penny and double it every day. This does not sound like it would amount to much, does it? You would have: $0.01, $0.02, $0.04, $0.08, $0.16, $0.32, $0.64, $1.28, $2.56, $5.12. On day ten, all you would have is $5.12. On day twenty, you would have $5,242. Day 25—$167,772. A nice chunk of change—but not filthy rich. But then, on day thirty—$5.37 million. During the first twenty-five days, change occurred relatively slowly. The last five days were really where most of the magic occurred. Lesson: it will often take some time before the real wonder manifests itself.

If you already enjoy a healthy lifestyle, kudos to you! However, if you don't, there is no need to fret. If you really want to make a change for the better, then the *decision* to do so is an important first step. More critical than the decision, though, is to take *action*. A decision made in your mind will not begin to change your life unless it is manifested in words and actions. Moreover, these actions should be small and consistent. You should take baby steps. It is my opinion that if you try to change your entire diet in a few days and transition from being a couch potato to running five miles within a week, you will be setting yourself up for failure.

Regarding diet, I believe that you should replace one unhealthy meal or snack a day with a healthy one. Do this every day for a week. Then replace a second unhealthy meal or snack with a healthy one for another week. Also, watch your portion sizes. We do not need to eat the contents of an entire plate that has food piled six inches high. Continue in this fashion, and over the course of a few weeks, you will find that your diet has changed markedly. Try to stick with foods that are in their most natural state possible—fresh fruits and vegetables, nuts, and grains. For extra motivation, you should realize that there is an abundance of resources—books, websites, and smartphone apps—available to teach you how to prepare healthy and tasty recipes. Moreover, a lot of the information found in digital formats is either free or accessible for a nominal fee.

As I mentioned, the same philosophy of baby steps applies to movement. I will preface this section with a disclaimer. If you have a medical condition, are under a doctor's care, or currently have a mostly sedentary lifestyle, then you should begin an exercise program with your doctor's approval and guidance. Having said that, humans were built to move. We were not meant to spend eight hours a day sitting in a cubicle, staring at a computer screen. Our brain, lungs, heart, muscles, and every other part of us needs to experience the joy of movement on a regular basis.

If you are not currently a very mobile individual, then start small. If you feel safe, take short walks around your neighborhood. You can do the same on a treadmill if you have access to one. Start with fifteen minutes at a leisurely pace. Do this a few times for a week. Next week, increase your walks to twenty minutes. Over the ensuing weeks, continue to increase both the time and the pace of your walks. Perhaps you will find yourself jogging after a while. You might also find that you want to engage in other physical activities, such as bicycling, swimming, strength training, yoga, Zumba, or organized sports.

Moreover, increasing the amount of moving that you do does not have to be a scheduled event. I am fairly certain that you may have heard this before, but I'll repeat it anyway. If you examine your day, I'll bet that you will find many opportunities for movement. For example, taking the stairs instead of the elevator, parking farther away from the store, doing calf raises while sitting at your desk, or even taking short breaks during your workday to stand up and stretch or maybe do a few push-ups or jumping jacks. There are likely numerous opportunities for movement that can be found in the nooks and crannies of your day, and it would be in your favor to take advantage of them. *Spoiler alert?—engaging in all this physical activity will cause you to feel fantastic! Not only will you appreciate this newfound euphoria, but so will your children, grandchildren, and other loved ones.*

Some people might be able to just jump right into a new physical routine and do well. However, I understand that it can frequently be difficult to get started. That is why taking baby steps is important. I realize that it is hard to get off a comfortable sofa and start moving on a consistent basis. I believe that the solution to this difficulty can be found in concepts that I learned about in my college physics class—inertia and momentum. My paraphrased definition of inertia is that a body at rest tends to remain at rest while a body in motion tends to remain in motion. Thus, if a body is at rest, it will resist movement. Conversely, if an object is moving, the tendency will be for it to continue doing so. Then comes the awesome power of momentum, which can be thought of as the energy gained by a moving object. I had an experience that I think illustrates this idea beautifully.

I run a few times each week, and I'll always remember one day, several years ago, when I went out for a run. Nothing out of the ordinary. However, for some reason, it seemed extremely difficult. My legs felt so tired. I felt the burn of lactic acid buildup early on. With each stride, I felt as though I wanted to stop. Maybe I just was not in the mood to run.

However, I kept going. I kept pushing through my desire to stop as well as the fatigue in my legs. I kept moving. After a short while, I no longer felt tired. It also didn't seem to require as much energy to keep my legs going. As a matter of fact, I was enjoying the feeling of my legs really pumping. My energy level continued to soar, and there was a point during my run when it felt as if I could continue for hours. When it was over, I felt great! Actually, some of the best and most intense workouts I've had have been on days when I was truly not in the mood to exercise.

I would like to briefly mention something equally important to movement—rest. Getting an adequate amount of sleep each night is essential for both your body and your mind. Although you might be quite busy, it is in your best interests to allow yourself a good night's sleep every day.

Takeaways

- Eat well most of the time. Keep the foods you eat as simple as possible. When preparing recipes, use wholesome ingredients.

- Consistency is key. Doing good things for yourself on a consistent basis will manifest as positive changes in your health and in the way you feel.
- Each of us is presented with choices every day. There are many beneficial things that you should opt to consume or partake in. By the same token, there are numerous things that should be avoided. Choose wisely.
- If your life and health both need a makeover, it does not have to happen overnight. This may very well be a setup for failure. Take things slowly. Heed the lesson taught to us by infants as they take one small step at a time until they find themselves joyously running around with huge smiles plastered across their faces.
- Also take note of the fact that when an infant falls during the time that they are learning to walk, they don't just sit there and decide it's not worth the effort. No matter how many times they fall, they will get up over and over and keep trying until they get it right. Otherwise, our streets would be filled with people crawling around.
- Sleep well each day.
- Move. Your body craves it.
- Always remember inertia and momentum. You are not the only one who feels lazy. We all do. That is, when we are still. When we have made the choice to change, and then commit to performing small actions on a consistent basis, the extraordinary power of momentum kicks in. The more you continue, the more momentum you will gain—which gets you going even more. It's a wonderful upward spiral. You will become unstoppable!

- The principles of choices, consistency, baby steps, inertia, and momentum do not only apply to eating and exercising. They apply to any goal you have set for yourself—whether it be related to health, sports, fitness, education, finances, career, or relationships. Momentum can help us do great things!

CHAPTER 8

FAILURE EQUALS OPPORTUNITY

Although understanding ideas such as baby steps, consistency, inertia, and momentum is important, it is also crucial to appreciate the fact that on whatever life journey you have chosen, there will be failures along the way. Some of these defeats will be on a smaller scale while others will be gargantuan. Although I realize that it may be difficult to do so in the moment, it is essential to view failures as learning opportunities.

Failures are wonderful chances to learn and grow. I'll bet that many of you know how to ride a bicycle. Do you remember when you were learning to ride? My first real bike was a Christmas gift from a man named Dave, who was my dad's boss when I was a kid. It was shiny red and came complete with a horn and training wheels. I can still recall how riding was a cinch with those training wheels. But that all changed when my dad took them off. Suddenly things became more complicated. A lot more complicated. Steering was now difficult, and I couldn't keep the bike straight. Maintaining my balance was even tougher, and I fell a lot. I had my battle wounds—lots of scrapes and bruises. However, each time I fell, my dad made me get back on the bike. Over time, my balance gradually improved, and I could ride in a straight line. Before I knew it, I was riding my bike well. Yippee! I was ecstatic. That was many years ago, and I still enjoy riding to this day. Thinking back on it, I would never have experienced the joy of riding if not for the many small failures and falls that taught me how to steer and keep my balance.

Fast-forward about ten years to just after high school. I was really excited about getting my license and being able to drive. I had my permit, and the day for my road test finally arrived. When I took the test for the first time (yes, there was a second time), I totally screwed up my parallel parking. I just couldn't get the angle right, and my tires kept hitting the curb. When I tried to indicate that I was going to pull out, the signal light did not start blinking. The windshield wipers turned on instead, and it took what seemed like an eternity for me to figure out how to shut them off. All this was happening while my instructor stared at me. When I finally got things straight and pulled out, I was directed to return to the location where the test began. I was so angry. I was not being given another chance to parallel park. I knew I had failed. I was so angry, in fact, that I really wasn't paying attention to the road on our way back. As I was about to make my final left turn, the car jerked to a halt. *What happened? Why did my instructor stop the car?* I was about to make a left turn into oncoming traffic. At that point, I knew I had really messed up.

I exited the vehicle feeling despondent. However, I learned two critical lessons that day: First, do not make left turns into oncoming traffic. Second, always pay attention to the road because there can be serious consequences if you don't. Those failures became lessons that have remained with me as an adult driver, and they have served me well. By the way, in case you're wondering, I did pass my road test the second time around.

Jumping ahead more than a decade, I found myself preparing to take my oral board examination in emergency medicine. I had done well on the written board exam, but the oral boards were a different animal. Compared to answering questions with a pencil and paper, it is much more intimidating to have a seasoned physician giving you clinical scenarios and asking how you would take care of your patients. The test definitely generated anxiety. Several weeks later, when my score report finally arrived in the mail, I opened the envelope slowly. When I read the letter, my heart sank. I failed—not by much—but I did fail. I was disappointed because I felt that all my diligent preparation was for naught. I would have to take it over again.

I scheduled another test date and purchased my airline tickets (the test was administered in Chicago). I studied assiduously over the course of several months. Although I was a bit apprehensive when test day arrived, I felt prepared. I went through the exam more confidently than the first time. When the scores arrived in the mail, I was quite pleased to learn that I had passed. When I look back on this experience, it seems that, rather than a failure, it was an event that allowed me to become a better physician as a result. I not only discovered how to organize my thoughts more efficiently while taking care of several patients at once but also learned additional material that helped me provide better care to them.

A couple of years after I became a board-certified emergency medicine physician, when my experience with kidney cancer led me on a path of self-education and I began to understand the value of a healthy lifestyle, I had another realization. I needed to help spread this message of the importance of living a healthy life. About a year prior to my epiphany, I had learned of a health and nutrition company, and I joined on as a distributor in the hope of earning extra money. When my life changed in 2007, it seemed as though this was really going to be the perfect opportunity. I could earn extra income while helping people become healthier. I believed in the products and took them every day.

I attended a lot of meetings over the phone and via the internet. I studied the company's literature and read several books on becoming a good salesperson. I wanted to help improve lives. I spoke to many people—some who I knew and many who were cold calls. I even went door-to-door. (One day as I did this, I was approached by a police officer. Apparently, someone had called the cops on me. I was informed that unless one represents a religious organization or has a license to do so, solicitation is illegal. Oops. For a moment I thought he was going to give me a ticket. Luckily, he just told me to go home, so I packed up and left.)

I did this over the course of a few years. However, despite my efforts, I never sold much product. Moreover, although I really did not want to admit it, I frequently had this nagging thought in the back of my mind telling me that I should be doing something more than selling supplements and nutrition bars. I eventually knew that I needed to follow my heart, and I phased myself out. I believe in the products and still take them today, but I learned that selling them was not my true desire.

Eventually, I decided to put my message of healthy living in writing. I began penning articles for local newspapers on the subjects of health and personal development. I was pleased to learn that my writing was well received. At some point, I had the idea to write a book, and I pursued this endeavor with great passion. At the time of this writing, I have written and independently published two children's books that impart lessons of healthy living. I derive great joy from writing, and I am happy that life has led me to this place.

There is one other story on the subject of failure that I would like to share. This one has nothing to do with health. It has to do with flying. Yes, flying. I had an interest in learning to fly for some time—more specifically, learning to fly a helicopter. One day, I decided to take a flight lesson. Given that I am deathly afraid of heights, this seemed a bit counterintuitive. Nevertheless, I decided to do it anyway. I wanted to have the experience. My flight instructor was terrific, and using my hands and feet to control an aircraft eight hundred feet above sea level was exhilarating. Although I was still scared up there, I enjoyed my flight so much that I decided to sign up for further lessons, both in the air and on the ground, which was the didactic aspect of flight school.

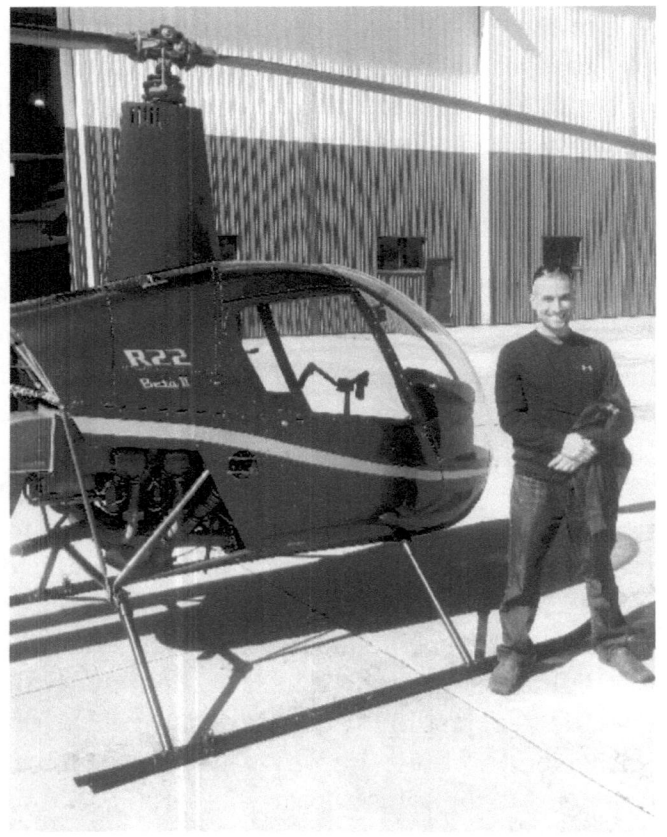

Me in flight school

One of the skills we practiced was hovering. It is quite challenging to coordinate the brain, hands, and feet to keep the aircraft in a hover, in one place, a few feet above the ground. I had been showing some improvement over the course of a few lessons. However, there was one lesson during which my flight instructor gave me greater reign over the controls, and I did much worse than I had in the past. In the moment, I felt disappointed with my performance. It wasn't until the drive home that I realized that my mistakes were vital for my learning and growth. My failures while learning to hover eventually helped me become more proficient at this skill.

Although this was a satisfying accomplishment, I came to realize that learning to fly a helicopter requires a great deal of time and effort. Besides the flying hours that are necessary to become a competent pilot, there is also an enormous amount of material that needs to be learned by reading and listening. Between working as a physician, writing, going to flight school, and enjoying time with my family, I felt as though I was stretching myself too thin. I began to appreciate the fact that I did not have the time for the commitment needed to become an excellent pilot. Moreover, becoming a mediocre pilot would be downright dangerous. I gave it a lot of thought and decided that I needed to give it up. It was a difficult yet necessary decision, and I have made peace with that choice. In addition, I don't view it as a loss but rather as a gain of many fantastic experiences, soaring through the air and seeing the world from a different perspective.

Takeaways

- Failure should not be considered a bad thing. As I mentioned earlier, it can sometimes be difficult to view failure as beneficial in the moment. If this is the case, you should give yourself some time to reflect on it afterward.

- Failures can be great teachers if we allow them to be. They can teach us the wrong way to do something. Moreover, if we can learn ten, twenty, or even a hundred or more incorrect ways to approach a task, we will have gained a wealth of experience and will be closer to figuring out the correct way to do it.
- Failures can help propel you forward. Repeated failures imply the presence of perseverance. They can be thought of as stepping-stones to success. It has been said that if you are not failing enough at something, then you are not trying hard enough.
- The most successful people in life are also the ones who have accumulated the most failures. For instance, do you know the following:
  - Thomas Edison is quoted as saying, "I have not failed. I've just found 10,000 ways that won't work."
  - James Dyson created 5,126 nonworking bagless vacuum prototypes. Prototype number 5,127 was the one that worked.
  - Michael Jordan was cut from his high school basketball team. He also said, "I've missed more than 9,000 shots in my career. I've lost almost 300 games. 26 times, I've been trusted to take the game winning shot and missed. I've failed over and over and over again in my life. And that is why I succeed."
  - Abraham Lincoln lost eight elections for various political offices.
  - Steve Jobs was forced out of the company he founded.

- o The wildly famous *Chicken Soup for the Soul* book series was initially rejected by 144 publishers.
- View failures as teachers and be persistent in your efforts. Never give up.
- Listen to your heart. If your feelings regarding a goal are mediocre at best, then perhaps it is not what you were put on this earth to do. However, if you have a true passion and excitement for something, you should persevere until you have accomplished that which you have set out to do.
- If you genuinely aspire to become exceptional at something, then you not only need to commit to it but also dedicate enough time to it. This may require you to turn down other commitments. Sometimes you need to say no, even to yourself.

CHAPTER 9

EXPANDING THE ZONE

Earlier, when I spoke about my junior high school days, I told the story of how I finally stood up to the hallway bullies. Although it was scary, it only took finding a few seconds of courage to stand up for myself. The fact that I can still clearly recall that incident so many years later tells me that it had a strong influence on me. I believe that it helped shape my life in a small, or perhaps a large, way. Remembering how frightened I was, I understand just how paralyzing the emotion of fear can be.

I have been afraid many times in my life. Looking back, I feel pride in the fact that many of those times, I pushed forward and did the thing that scared me. I suppose I have some courage. Courage, by the way, does not imply being fearless. It entails doing something despite being afraid. Sometimes it may only be necessary to be courageous one time in order to conquer a fear; other occasions require that courage be exercised many times to develop a level of comfort.

As an older adolescent, I was very much a bodybuilding enthusiast. Although I have a small frame, I really enjoyed pumping iron. I loved doing bicep curls, bench presses, squatting, shoulder presses, and a host of other exercises. I loved the burn and the feeling of being pumped (I still thrive on these sensations). During that time, I had learned about supplements that were supposed to enhance muscle building. These came in the form of a few pills that I took religiously. Until I didn't.

One day, things changed. I was sitting on the sofa in my basement and put one of the pills in my mouth. I raised a glass of water to my lips, took a gulp, and swallowed. This time something went wrong. The pill did not go down smoothly. It got stuck. I could feel it in the back of my throat. I could not get it to go down, so I began to panic. I drank more water. Still stuck. I remember thinking, *What if it doesn't go down?* What seemed like an hour probably lasted less than twenty seconds. I swallowed hard and drank more water. My panic rose to frightening levels. Then, finally, the pill passed. I was so relieved.

Initially, I thought that this was going to be an isolated event. However, the next time I went to take my supplements, I found that I couldn't. I would put the pill in my mouth and try to drink water, but I could not seem to coordinate the actions of moving the pill to the back of my mouth and drinking the water. I tried a few more times. *Place pill in mouth, drink, and swallow.* Unsuccessful. Initially, I thought that something was physically wrong with me. Then I realized that I was actually afraid to move the pill to the back of my mouth and swallow it. I had just developed a phobia of swallowing pills.

I believe that I made a few more attempts on different days to take my supplements, but to no avail. At some point, I made the decision that I was not going to take any more pills. I had a new fear that I carried with me for almost two decades. I knew that it was irrational. I mean, when I ate, I swallowed pieces of food that were larger than some of the pills I had been taking. No problem there. Nevertheless, I could not bring myself to take another pill. I was ashamed of it, and for a long time, I never mentioned it to anyone.

When I became interested in the nutritional supplement company in 2006, I found myself in a dilemma. I wanted to use the company's products. But they were pills, and I was afraid to take pills. I didn't know what to do, so I finally decided to ask for help. I told Mayra about my phobia of swallowing pills, and she helped me work through my fear. Yes, she was able to explain the actual steps one needs to take when swallowing a pill. However, it was much more than that. Just knowing that somebody else, especially a person I knew well and trusted, was supporting me proved to be a huge benefit.

As I recall, it did not happen overnight but rather over several weeks. I started out with supplements that were small tablets, yet I was still afraid of them getting stuck in the back of my throat. I worked through the motion slowly and consistently, until finally, one day, I experienced success. I had swallowed a small tablet. I gradually forged ahead and began to take larger, capsule-shaped pills. Over time, I became quite a good pill taker. I realize that this may seem like a trivial thing to many, but it was very real in my mind. Furthermore, I cannot overstate just how helpful it was to have Mayra in my corner. It is said that necessity is the mother of invention. I learned that necessity might also be just the impetus one needs to overcome fears.

Conquering this fear when I started out in the supplement business was a great accomplishment. I had most certainly grown as a result. During my time attempting to sell supplements, I also expanded myself in another way. As mentioned in an earlier chapter, one of the things I did to promote the product I was selling was to make cold calls. This essentially means calling total strangers and pitching your product to them. I found that this is not an easy thing to do. I could think of a ton of reasons not to pick up the phone. *What if they're busy? What if they're in the middle of something important? What if they have no interest in vitamins? What if they have no interest in their health? What if they just don't want to be bothered?* So many reasons not to make the call and only a single reason to pick up the phone—to try to show the person at the other end of the line how my product could add value to their life.

At the outset, I felt considerable trepidation each time I was about to dial a number. I could feel my heart thumping in my chest. When someone picked up, I often stumbled over my words. Many people hung up right away. Some listened for a few minutes before I heard the dreaded click. Others stayed on the phone awhile, seemed interested, and asked that I get back to them. For the most part, I always got a voice mail when I called back at the scheduled time and never heard from them again. Then there were a few people with whom I had long conversations and really got into giving them some advice on issues they were dealing with.

Although all this cold calling did not help me sell more supplements, it did help me to stretch myself in new ways. I moved well out of my comfort zone and gained confidence while becoming more at ease trying to persuade a stranger to try a product that might prove to be of benefit to them. Moving out of one's comfort zone is exceedingly important for growth.

Speaking of comfort zones, mine is, for the most part, on the ground. I mentioned earlier that I am quite fearful of heights. Yes, I know I went to flight school for a short time and trained to fly a helicopter. That absolutely required some courage. However, for some reason, I am not as scared if I'm in an aircraft. But try to get me to stand by the edge of a cliff—I'm sorry, but that's just not going to happen.

Although I won't stand at the end of a precipice, I do enjoy being out in nature. One of the things I love is hiking. Being outside and experiencing the serenity of a forest, valley, or mountain is wonderful. Breathing in clean air that carries the scent of the surrounding trees is remarkably refreshing. Beholding lush green vistas from atop a mountain is incredible. It's easy to want to sit there for hours and take it all in. I thoroughly enjoy doing this, and as long as I am a safe distance from an edge, I am comfortable. There have been a few instances, though, during which I've missed out on some amazing things because I was too afraid to move into uncharted territory.

A few years ago, my family and I took a trip to Utah. It is an incredible place. The towering red-rock mountains were amazing. We visited several national parks while we were there and did a ton of hiking and exploring. It's a trip I'll likely never forget. Specifically, there is one part of our adventure that I will definitely never forget. One day, we visited Arches National Park in the city of Moab. This place is nothing short of spectacular. It is filled with two thousand massive rocky arches, many looming high over surrounding canyons. One particular arch is considered to be the most famous of all—Delicate Arch. If you've seen pictures of arches from this park, chances are that you've seen Delicate Arch.

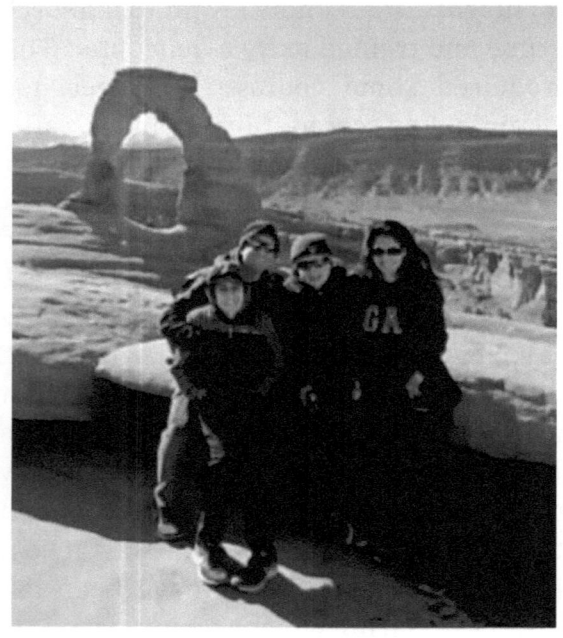

My family and Delicate Arch

During our day at the park, we did the hike up to Delicate Arch. It was an exhilarating trek that required some effort. Once we got closer to the end, it was obvious that our hard work was well worth it. There it was. Delicate Arch stood so proudly and gracefully not too far off in the distance, and we admired the view. To my great surprise, the hike was not yet over. Apparently, you can walk right up to Delicate Arch and appreciate it while standing directly under it. This would be breathtaking. Or so I thought.

We had to climb over a small rocky wall a few feet high and ended up on the curved and slightly downward-sloping rim of a canyon. A short walk along this rim would take us to the arch. No problem. Mayra and our younger son, Joey, went ahead, stood by the arch, and took photographs. My older son, Josh, who is also afraid of heights, stayed with me. I tried to encourage Josh to walk over to the arch. The problem came after I took a few steps and froze. My muscles tensed, and I could not move. I became acutely aware of just how high up I was and could see myself slipping and rolling down the rim into the canyon below. Please note that we were walking on a rather wide rim; it certainly was not a balancing act. Nevertheless, I could not get myself to move forward.

Mayra and Joey returned from their adventure at the arch. She then took Josh to cross over to it. Joey, who was eleven at the time, stayed with me. Josh did fantastically. Despite being scared, he walked across the rim and stood by the arch. I was so proud of him. My story, on the other hand, was quite a bit different. I could no longer stand, and I sat down with my back snug against the small rocky wall along the outside of the rim. Joey extended his hand and tried to help me, but I would not move. I was terrified. My heart was beating wildly, and I didn't know what to do. I needed to get back over the rocky wall to the other side—the safer side. The trouble was that I was too afraid to even move. What a quandary—I needed to get up to escape danger but was too afraid to move. Joey, who started out in helping mode, began laughing hysterically. "Just get up," he said with a big smile.

"I can't move," I said.

This went on for a few minutes. Another problem was that I had my backpack on, and I was afraid I would lose my balance while wearing it, causing me to roll into the canyon and fall to my death. Mind you, the backpack really was not too heavy. I told Joey about my backpack issue, and he told me to give it to him. So I did just that. I gave the backpack, the one that I feared would cause me to lose my balance and fall, to my eleven-year-old son. Pretty brave of me, right? I was at the point where I knew I had to do something. Finally, I mustered up a few seconds of courage, grabbed Joey's hand, and pulled myself up. I quickly turned and climbed over the rocky wall that I had been sitting against. What a sigh of relief I breathed. I was thankful that Joey was there to help me, even though he was still laughing at me.

Mayra, Josh, and Joey all have pictures of themselves standing next to Delicate Arch. I do not have such a picture. Perhaps if I had had more time to acclimate myself better, I would have walked over to the arch. I can't say for certain. I did miss out on this experience because I feared leaving my comfort zone, but I decided to be OK with this choice. However, as illustrated from some of my other experiences, I strongly believe that it is important to move out of your comfort zone when it involves something that will enable you to improve your life.

Although fear is a powerful emotion, it can be overcome. It may not be easy, but it can be done. Moreover, sometimes other people can motivate us to conquer our fear. Mayra was there for me when I defeated my fear of swallowing pills. Another instance found Josh as my motivator. Several years ago, while on another vacation, we visited a water park in Florida. We passed by the cliff-diving attraction, and it seemed like it would be fun. It did not look too high, and there also happened to be no line, so we decided to give it a try. Josh and I walked to the top of the "cliff." I had been prepared to jump first—until we got to the top and looked down. It looked much higher from our new vantage point than it did from the ground.

We stood up there for a few minutes, both trying to be brave. Each of us was saying how we would jump first, yet neither of us made a move. I was beginning to feel like quite the chicken up there when Josh unexpectedly jumped into the pool below. Boy, was I surprised. I was also proud. At this point, I had no choice. My son had just jumped, which meant that I had to do the same. After a few deep breaths, I took a step forward and jumped into the pool below. I was scared for a few seconds before I splashed into the water, after which I felt exhilarated. We went back to do it a second time, and then a third. We probably spent nearly an hour jumping off that cliff, and if it hadn't been for Josh, I may never have jumped at all.

What began as an anxiety-provoking experience ended up being a fantastic time. Thinking back on it, I was most anxious before I jumped, before I really knew what to expect. Once I had done it, my anxiety levels plummeted. Many times we are afraid of the unknown, and once the mysterious becomes familiar, our anxiety dissipates.

I can recall similar experiences during public speaking events. My first real experience with public speaking came at the end of junior high school. I was the class salutatorian, which meant that I had to deliver a speech at graduation. I can remember standing on the stage behind the podium, staring at hundreds of faces. The sheet of paper containing my speech was shaking uncontrollably in my hands. My heart was pounding against my chest, and I kept worrying that people were going to get bored during my talk. I did finish my speech, and I believe it was good. Jumping ahead to college, I decided to take a public speaking class, and I did rather well. However, the final talk for that class was more of a challenge than I had anticipated. I was discussing home aquariums, and my best friend decided it was a good time to have some fun with me. He kept pressing his face up against the small glass window in the door and making weird expressions. He was directly to my right, and I was the only one who could see him. I was forced to concentrate that much harder to remain focused on my topic and refrain from laughing. Over the subsequent decades, I have had the opportunity to speak in front of many audiences. Although I still do get nervous at times, I have become much more at ease while speaking in public.

Takeaways

- Many people enjoy staying in their comfort zone because it is in this place where they feel most, well, comfortable. It's nice to be comfortable, to know what to expect. Moving out of this place can induce anxiety and fear. There is the fear of failure. Remember, failures should be viewed as opportunities for learning and growth and are thus good things.
- There is also the fear of embarrassment. Nobody wants to make a fool of themselves. It can be difficult to put yourself out there and risk getting laughed at. If this is indeed a concern, you should ask yourself if what you are venturing to do is going to make you happy. If it is, then just go for it. In the end, it is not other people who are going to bring you true happiness. You are the only person who can do that. It's OK to fail in front of others. Perhaps you might experience embarrassment, but that's a temporary emotion. The important thing is that you have just learned another way not to do something. Furthermore, there may be someone in your presence who knows how to do that which you are attempting to learn.
- The definition of courage is not being fearless but instead moving forward despite your fear. Always move forward. Expand yourself. Employ the support offered by others. Consider failures to be the stepping-stones to your success. Allow your comfort zone to stretch. You will be a better person because of it.

CHAPTER 10

The Little Things

In your journey to enlarge your comfort zone, and regarding life in general, always be cognizant of the fact that many times the small things matter. In fact, it is the consistent small actions that will bring about tremendous results. Recall that these results, depending on the choices that have been made over time, can be good or bad. However, for now, I want to focus on the good. I mentioned this concept earlier when I told the story of the magic penny, but I'd like to briefly touch on it again.

What exactly are the small things when it comes to being healthy? Choosing an apple instead of a cookie. A glass of water rather than a soda. Broccoli instead of french fries. A protein-packed quinoa-and-bean salad rather than a cheeseburger. Going for a walk instead of lounging on the couch. Jogging instead of surfing the internet. Going to the gym (or working out at home) instead of watching prime-time television.

To be clear, the importance of small, consistent actions does not only apply to health. It applies to pretty much everything in life. Do you want to excel in your career? If so, do something each day at work to benefit your team. Do you wish to become a better baseball player? Get out there and practice on most days. Do you want to increase your savings? Each time you get paid, be sure to pay yourself first and put that money into the bank or a retirement account. Are you falling in love and wish to spend the rest of your life with that special someone? Do something each day that shows how much you care.

Expressing love and kindness through repeated small gestures most certainly has a positive compounding effect over time. Making coffee each morning for my wife puts a smile on her face and creates closeness between us. I can sense my boys' appreciation when I graciously help them with their homework. During every occasion when I take the time to be present and listen at the bedside while my patients speak, I can feel their gratefulness. When somebody holds the door for me, or I encounter a friendly clerk at the supermarket checkout counter, it inspires me to be the same way toward others.

Although they don't seem like much in the moment, over time, the little things most definitely matter. Small adjustments lead to huge changes. This fact was also demonstrated to me through martial arts. I studied tae kwon do for about a year before attending medical school. I loved it, but I stopped when medical school started. Many years later, I enrolled in a different tae kwon do school with my family. After a couple of years, I suffered a knee injury requiring surgery and ended up leaving the school. During that time, I met a man who was a longtime martial artist and self-defense expert. He started offering self-defense lessons a few times each week.

His classes were attended by a small group of people, and he taught us some amazing things. For example, he showed us how to escape headlocks (I wish I had learned this about thirty-five years ago). He taught us how to step and turn to escape the hold. It is actually a simple move. However, when it was initially taught to me, I was unable to free myself from the hold. My instructor then told me to change the angle of the direction in which I was stepping. It was quite a small change, and I didn't think that it would make much of a difference. I tried it and—voilà—I escaped! I was astounded by how such a tiny change in the way I stepped enabled me to break free of a headlock. When considering just how incredibly significant small changes are, it turns out that martial arts are a microcosm of life in general.

Takeaways

- Pay attention to the small things. Small, simple, and seemingly unimportant decisions will weigh in heavily over the years.
- Make choices that will work in your favor over the long term. The choices you make each day in the present will directly affect all aspects of your life in the future.

CHAPTER 11

WILLPOWER? NOT SO MUCH

Making good choices every day is essential to one's general health and well-being. Of course, there needs to be a conscious effort involved in making these decisions, and sometimes it may be difficult to make good ones. This is where the power of building habits enters the picture. This involves choosing to perform a duty or task on a regular basis. As I mentioned, this may be burdensome at first. However, over time, the behaviors will become automatic. Once this automaticity kicks in, the behaviors will be performed with ease. They will become something you do without thought.

For instance, I had read somewhere that performing some form of physical activity immediately upon rousing from bed can really help wake you up and get you ready for your day. I decided to give it a try and chose to do twenty-five repetitions of an abdominal exercise called bicycles first thing in the morning. Initially, the required mental effort was slightly tough. However, after doing this for perhaps a week or so, it became second nature. Getting out of bed equaled doing twenty-five bicycles, and it really did help me feel more awake.

Pairing a new behavior with something you already do can also help you build a routine of regularly performing that activity. Perhaps you want to do ten push-ups each day. You could begin doing five push-ups twice daily. Once in the morning and once at night—right before you brush your teeth. Toothbrushing will equal five push-ups.

Developing healthy eating habits is also not that difficult. However, just as with most other endeavors, it does require some commitment and discipline. Perhaps you could start eating a nutritious daily midmorning snack. Grapes, carrots, and nuts are all great options. Do it each day and it will soon become second nature. If you order an unhealthy take-out lunch every day at work, begin packing your own more wholesome lunch the night before. This not only will likely save you money but also the small investment of your time will have big payoffs in the future. Expand on this. Work with each meal. Replace unhealthy ones with healthy ones. Initially, this will require effort. Over time, though, the practice will develop into a habit and become easier and easier. Remember momentum? It will soon become obvious that the self-destructive habits that you may have can eventually be replaced by good ones.

Cigarette smoking is also an example that comes to mind. Let me preface this by saying that I have never been a smoker and that I am not an expert on smoking cessation. However, I believe that if you develop a craving for a cigarette, you can do something else to take your mind off that yearning. Examples include chewing a piece of gum or going for a brisk walk.

One additional point worth mentioning is willpower. Many may feel that willpower is necessary to make changes and build up the routines outlined in these paragraphs. My opinion is that this is true but only to a small degree. I have both read about and experienced how it can be exhausting to use willpower all the time. Trying to avoid unhealthy foods that you enjoy so that you can begin eating more nutritious foods that you will also enjoy can be tough. Rather than exercising willpower, the better solution is to avoid temptation.

Several years ago, Mayra taught religious education to elementary schoolchildren at a school affiliated with our local church. During the last class before Christmas break, many of the students approached her bearing gifts. There were scented candles, ornaments, candied apples, and candy. These were thoughtful gestures, and we were grateful.

The candy sat on our kitchen counter over the ensuing weeks, and its quantity steadily dwindled. Although I do not eat sweets on a regular basis, I did partake in some chocolates on several occasions. They were delicious, and I really enjoyed them. I'm sure that by now you are well aware that I eat healthy foods most of the time. I thus believe that it is fine to enjoy treats once in a while. Because of this, I indulge without regret.

However, during these weeks, with the candy resting on our countertop, I came to a realization. I understood that I would not have eaten any candy at all had it not been there in the first place. With easy access to unhealthy treats, using willpower becomes quite difficult if temptation is staring you in the face. Therefore, if you are sincerely trying to become a healthier, more vibrant person, it would behoove you to rid your kitchen pantry and cupboards of unhealthy foods. Just as important is keeping it well stocked with nutritious foods. This will ensure that you have access to only healthy ingredients with which to prepare meals. Furthermore, when those cravings for a snack begin, you can rest assured that you will not be reaching for junk food.

Takeaways

- The routines that you develop for yourself will keep you in line with where you want to be in life. Realize that, although it may be difficult at first, the future payoffs will be well worth your efforts.
- The choices you make today will have an enormous effect on your future self. Do you wish for your future self to have an easy or a difficult life? Do you want your future self to be healthy and vibrant or unhealthy and fatigued?
- Please also appreciate that if you truly desire change, you will find that you do have the discipline to begin building new habits. If your aspiration is strong enough, you will manifest the necessary effort and discipline. In other words, if your *why* is powerful, the *how* will reveal itself.
- While building your new habits, don't rely solely on willpower to avoid urges. Remove temptation from the outset. You will find that it will make your journey much easier.

CHAPTER 12

CURVEBALLS

You have committed to making better, healthier choices. Over time, your life will improve because of it. However, you must realize that, although you are doing things to improve yourself, many things in life are still not within your control. No matter how disciplined you are, unexpected circumstances are going to occur. Yes, life is going to throw you curveballs.

These unanticipated events will show up in many ways. You are about to go out for a run and a heavy downpour begins. You have set time aside to go to the gym and someone from work calls with an urgent need for your expertise. You are about to start preparing a healthy recipe, only to learn that you are missing a key ingredient. Your teenage son just hit a baseball and broke a window. Your car gets a flat while on the way to an important meeting. Your flight is delayed. You have a disagreement with your spouse that is about to lead to a huge argument.

Yes, there will be lots of curveballs that we have absolutely no control over. However, the really great thing to remember is that we *do have control over how we respond* to these unforeseen events. That decision is entirely ours. What happens to us is not as important as how we respond to these situations. Notice also that I said *respond* rather than *react*. I think of reacting as more like a knee-jerk reflex that occurs without much conscious thought. You know what I'm talking about. You're running late and traffic suddenly slows to a crawl. Many times, we, myself included, would instantly get angry and stressed. We may curse and smack the steering wheel. That is an example of reacting. However, in that small segment of time when we realize that we are about to be stuck in traffic, we have a choice. We have the ability to take a step back and choose. We can react and allow anger to overcome us and swear aloud, or we can respond and take a deep breath, realizing that the traffic is out of our control. We can sit back, relax, enjoy some good music, and just be present in the moment.

It is within that small expanse of time that our power lies. We can either decide to react with fury or to respond with understanding. That choice is ours. We don't have to yell at our child when the baseball flies through the window. We can tell him to be more careful and be grateful that nobody was harmed. We can decide to fully listen to our spouse's perspective instead of becoming defensive. We can choose to do a workout indoors if there is torrential rain outside. If that key ingredient is missing, we can take a few minutes to research some other options using what we do have available in our kitchen. If a project we've been working on is suddenly derailed, we can pause and brainstorm ways to get back on track. Perhaps ideas will surface that will make our project better than it was.

It is clear from these examples that flexibility is a vital trait to have. Things will change, and being flexible will allow us to adjust and keep moving forward, perhaps even improving our original objective. This idea brings to mind palm trees. Palm trees are beautiful. Have you ever seen palm trees during a storm? They bend in the wind. Their flexibility prevents them from snapping when confronted with a gale. This is one reason why they flourish in tropical climates, where there is no shortage of high-wind storms. Flexibility also calls to mind skyscrapers. These colossal structures are engineered to be pliable to a certain degree. This will help prevent them from collapsing during earthquakes and other natural disasters.

Sometimes when the unanticipated happens and we react, anger may not be the predominant emotion that wells up in our minds. We may instead experience anxiety. I remember one such moment clearly. On October 29, 2011, I was scheduled to work the night shift in the ER. That also happened to be the day when we had the first big snowstorm of the season, and I found myself having to drive to work in the heavy snowfall. I was already in a bit of a hurry because I wanted to leave home earlier than usual. Anyone who was driving that evening knew that the roads were in extremely poor condition. The traffic was not cooperating either. I was at a complete standstill for close to an hour. I soon realized that, in my haste, I had forgotten to take my knapsack, which held my hospital ID, my stethoscope, and a few other work essentials. I also found myself in need of a toilet. These problems were running through my mind for a while. I was becoming quite anxious because I was worried about being late and not having my "doctor gear."

Before long, I recognized that my apprehension was not going to change anything. It certainly wasn't going to make me get to work any faster. So I took a deep breath and decided to stop worrying. The rest of the ride was much more serene. Yes, I was an hour late, but the ER was not too busy. It so happened that one of my colleagues lent me her stethoscope. I survived the shift just fine.

This story illustrates one example of worry that evolved into anxiety. Unfortunately, this is an emotion with which I am familiar. I have suffered from anxiety since I was a child, and I understand what a powerful emotion it can be. I can recall episodes of anxiety as a child, as a teenager, and as an adult during medical school. A common theme of these experiences was feeling as though I was being closed in. There was a vague yet powerful sense of impending doom, with nowhere to turn for help. To be candid, it was terrifying.

Anxiety may arise due to unexpected circumstances, or it may just become a part of daily life. For the most part, I am fortunate to experience anxiety only on rare occasions (such as when I know I am going to be really late for work). For myself, I find that taking a few deep breaths and stepping back from the situation is extremely helpful. Disclaimer: I am not a therapist or professionally qualified to treat anxiety. However, I really believe that the simple act of becoming cognizant of my breathing and consciously trying to slow it down provides a lot of relief. Believe me, I also realize that this is so much easier said than done. Nevertheless, that does not imply that it can't be done. With conscious and consistent effort, solace from anxiety might just be attained. Along these lines, I would like to briefly mention meditation. I was introduced to this practice after my cancer diagnosis. I have become familiar with two types of meditation practice, mindfulness and transcendental. Although I am not a meditation expert, I would highly recommend learning and practicing meditation. There is a wealth of resources on the subject available, and as I find that it helps bring calmness and clarity to my life, it can to yours too.

"Can any of you by worrying add a single moment to your life-span?" (Matthew 6:27, New American Bible, Revised Edition.) Whether you are a person of faith or not, I believe that these words of Jesus are timeless and true.

Takeaways

- Flexibility is important. If something unexpected occurs, being flexible goes hand in hand with responding rather than reacting. You have that capability. We all do.
- There will always be that small moment in time between when you become aware that circumstances have changed and you are presented with a choice. Will you react or respond? Will you respond and be flexible, or react and be rigid?

- Depending on the circumstances, sometimes responding and being flexible will force you to change your perspective, thus allowing you to come up with ideas that you might not have thought of had the unexpected not occurred.
- If you find yourself feeling anxious, closing your eyes and taking a few slow and deep breaths may prove helpful in bringing about calm.

CHAPTER 13

PERSPECTIVES

Anxiety and anger can be strong emotions. Of course, they can certainly be bad things. However, it's important to realize that our emotions are frequently the result of our perceptions. The manner in which we see a situation is our perspective. The serene weather within the eye of a hurricane is in stark contrast to the violent winds and torrential rains that comprise the rest of the storm. Thus, depending on which part of the storm you happen to be in (your perspective), the environment will be quite different. As a practitioner of medicine, I have an entirely different perspective than a layperson. The sudden onset of abdominal pain will likely have a different meaning for me than for, let's say, an astrophysicist. It would be as though I am on a totally different level of understanding with regard to the situation. Similarly, if there was some enormous cosmic event that was going to impact our Earth, the converse would be true. The astrophysicist would have an understanding that I could probably not even fathom.

We have a six-year-old yellow Labrador retriever named Rocky. For a while after he first arrived in our home, I thought that I knew a lot about owning and raising dogs. Not so. Rocky was beginning to display behavioral issues that we were concerned about, and I didn't know what to do. Around that time, I happened to come across a copy of *Cesar's Way*, by dog behavior expert Cesar Millan. Mr. Millan taught me a completely different way to view canine behavior. I learned how dogs see the world. I gained a new perspective, and it helped a great deal. (Prior to the behavioral issues, Mayra had already read one of Mr. Millan's books and watched a few episodes of his television show and had mentioned some of his ideas to me. I, of course, did not listen at the time. She, of course, was right. I should have listened.)

Proper perspective is essential, as it can help in all life situations. It can be especially valuable under stressful circumstances. When these situations arise, take a step back and ask yourself if there is any other way to look at things. Using the example of being stuck in traffic, the way in which you *respond* to this situation can depend on your perspective. If you see this solely as a situation that is going to make you late, anger may very well be the first emotion that surfaces. Conversely, if you view the crawling traffic as providing you with some extra time to relax and unwind, it may be tranquility that you experience.

How about this suggestion? If you are truly stuck awhile with no immediate hope for an alternate route, try to perceive the situation as one in which you have some extra time for yourself. After all, this circumstance is out of your control, and no matter what is going on in your head, be it rage or peacefulness, it is going to have zero effect on moving the traffic along any faster. Thus, you might as well make the best of things by being kind to yourself and enjoying the solitude.

Another thing to consider in the event of a traffic jam is not only *changing* your perspective but also *broadening* your perspective. Try to think outside of just yourself. After all, why is there traffic in the first place? Did somebody's car break down? If so, they are likely having a more difficult day than you. Even worse, was there an accident? Did somebody suffer serious harm or perhaps lose their life? Thinking about such possibilities makes being angry because you are stuck in traffic seem trivial. Just like everything else that we have control over, we have a choice about how we perceive the world around us. It took me several decades to realize this, but I'm glad that I can finally appreciate this truth.

Perspective is important not only when dealing with external events but also when dealing with other people. We all have filters, or lenses, through which we see the world around us. I can remember working a shift in the ER that ended at 11:00 p.m. It had been a busy day, and one of my last patients was a young woman in her thirties. Per the nurse's notes in the chart, she had come to the ER with complaints of chronic abdominal pain and constipation. After reading that, a barrage of thoughts flooded my mind:

Did this patient come here just to receive narcotic pain medications?

Is she lying about her pain?

It's almost the end of my shift. Why did she come here so late at night with a complaint of constipation?

Almost immediately, my perception of her was distorted. I had not yet exchanged even a single word with her, but I already had thoughts about the type of person she was. I was seeing her through cloudy lenses.

However, I decided to approach her as I do every patient—with kindness and an open mind. I spoke with her at length and learned a bit about her. It turned out that she was a genuinely warmhearted individual who was going through some difficult times. I tried to figure out the best way to help her. Moreover, she declined any offer of pain medications. All my initial perceptions were incorrect.

We all encounter people in a host of different locations and situations. It is often quite easy to prejudge other individuals without ever giving them an opportunity to express who they are, what they are feeling, or what kind of day they are having. Have you ever encountered an unpleasant and impatient cashier at the checkout counter of your local supermarket? I would propose that instead of acting in a similar fashion, you broaden your perspective and look at that individual through clean lenses. Perhaps they have a sick child at home. Maybe their car just broke down. Perhaps they don't have enough money to buy food for their family. Or maybe they *are* just grumpy all the time. In any case, a little kindness on your part can go a long way to brighten that person's day.

A concept related to living life with clean lenses is appreciating the fact that our mind's principal job is to protect us from all threats, both physical and emotional. I'm sure that you have experienced this instinct many times. I know that I have and continue to do so on occasion. For instance, if Mayra and I are having a discussion that is evolving into a disagreement, she may make a statement that opposes a belief I have. Thoughts will then arise in my mind about how wrong she is. I will make statements to myself such as *She doesn't know what she is talking about*, and I will ask myself questions such as *Why would she say that to me?* Even if we share the same goal, I will become internally upset if she doesn't see my way as the correct way.

I have learned that I experience these feelings because my beliefs are being challenged. My mind's job is to protect me, and if someone tells me that my opinions are wrong, that is a high-threat situation. These feelings float around in my mind, and I am aware of them as well as the associated emotions of anger and shame. When these feelings and emotions do emerge, I am presented with two choices, as you may have already guessed. I can either react to them or respond to them. The decision is entirely mine. If I react, there is likely going to be a heated argument. If I respond, things will play out much differently. The emotions will still be there, and I can allow them to be there. However, I can decide to be open-minded and listen to what Mayra has to say. Perhaps she is right (as she usually is). Maybe I will learn something from the experience (as I often do). Responding will allow us to have a thoughtful and respectful exchange of ideas that will be beneficial to both of us.

In short, when facing your own heated discussions, and given that there is likely no immediate threat to your well-being, know that you have the capability to have a polite exchange of ideas. You will not always be right, and that's perfectly fine. We are all human and being wrong does not make you any less so.

Takeaways

- Proper perspective is essential, especially in difficult situations. It can be incredibly worthwhile to take a step back and ask yourself if there is any other way to look at things.
- Seek advice. Read an article or book. Many times, the perspective of others can be a wonderful gift, helping to provide the enlightenment needed to assist us in solving many of life's challenging quandaries.
- When it comes to other people, unless it is clear that they are intentionally trying to do you harm, you should give them the benefit of the doubt. You likely have no idea what the involved person is going through in life. Before you venture out into the world each day, please be sure to clean off your lenses.
- It is OK to have disagreements. Polite dialogues can still occur in the context of differences, and perhaps one or more participants will learn something new.

CHAPTER 14

VANTAGE POINTS

I would like to spend a little more time discussing perspective. However, I would like to discuss this concept in terms of seeing our own internal lives from different vantage points. Many times, we may become so engrossed in the current state of affairs of our lives that we are unable to see anything else. Imagine if you could step out of your body and view your life from a mile away. What would it look like? Would you see anything that you are just not able to see because you are literally right in the middle of things? Would you come to gain a new understanding and develop new ideas?

There was one day a couple of summers ago that was filled with errands. For whatever reason, I had quite a long to-do list and everything on it needed to be completed that day. I had been driving from place to place, checking off items as I went. Things had been going smoothly. However, when late afternoon arrived, I still found myself with many tasks that had not yet been completed. I was becoming impatient and somewhat overwhelmed as I felt myself rushing to my next errand. *I'm never going to be able to get all this done.* As I drove, my negative emotions grew stronger. Then it happened. I'm not sure how it occurred, but it did. A profound sense of calm overcame me. Suddenly the number of remaining items on my list didn't matter. I somehow knew that I would get everything done and that there was no need to rush. I realized that the rest of the day was going to go smoothly, and it did.

This experience, although unintentional, almost did feel as though I was suddenly viewing myself from a different perspective. It was surreal, but in a good way. Something allowed me to see myself as tranquil and having lots of time rather than anxious and almost out of time. The message that I took away from that day was that I have the ability to consciously perform the same shift in perspective when circumstances appear to be getting out of hand.

As it relates to perspective and vantage points, I also believe that our lives are composed of many potential levels and that it is up to us to ascend these levels to grow as a person. My thoughts drift to dogs and children as good illustrations of this concept.

Dogs are typically loyal, playful, and lovable creatures. Besides Rocky, we also have an apricot miniature poodle named Buddy and our newest addition, Bailey, who is a golden retriever. While Rocky loves tug-of-war, Buddy's game of choice is fetch. Currently, it seems that one of Bailey's favorite activities is chewing on shoes. Yes, they all have their moments of mischievousness—chewing on our furniture, walls, and floor, stealing food off the countertops, and so on. Nonetheless, they are true members of our family. There are days when Mayra and I are both working and our sons are at school. As I am leaving in the morning on these days, all three gaze at me with sad eyes. I feel terrible leaving them for the day, yet I am an adult with responsibilities and a career. Believe it or not, I tell them where I am going. I apologize for leaving and provide assurance that I will see them later in the day.

I feel confident that, on some level, they understand what I am feeling. However, I am fairly certain that they are unable to appreciate the fact that I go to work to help earn money for the household. Although dogs are quite intelligent, I do not believe they are able to grasp concepts such as money, career, and expenses. These notions are above their level of reasoning.

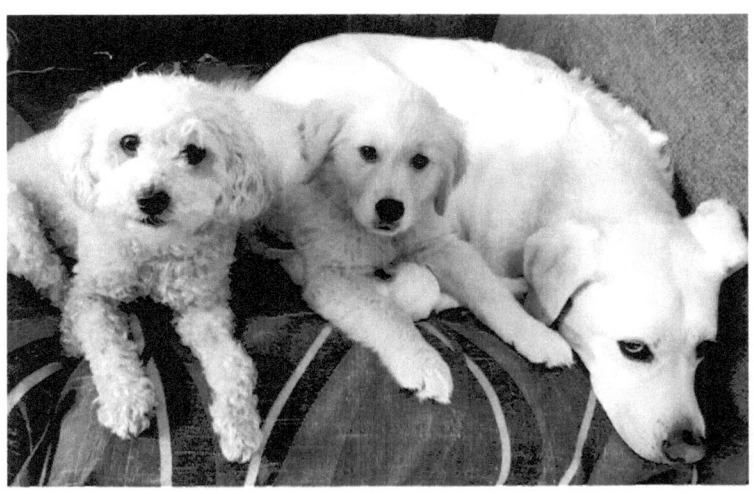

Our furry babies

All creatures capable of thought have some degree of intelligence. The extent of intelligence and understanding not only varies widely among sentient beings but also fluctuates based on the individual's age. I hold many clear memories of my boys as infants and toddlers. I have recollections of early steps, bedtime stories, spoon-feeding them baby food (much of it was rather tasty), playtime in their toy house, and crayoned pictures on our walls (between the dogs and the kids, our walls have been through a lot).

Back in 2007, when I received my cancer diagnosis, it was a trying time for both Mayra and me. While there were instances when I feared that I might not survive to see my boys grow up, all Josh and Joey knew was that Daddy had a boo-boo. Terms such as *cancer*, *surgery*, and *chemotherapy* were foreign to them. *Boo-boo* was the extent of their understanding. It was all they were capable of at the time; anything else was above their level of thought.

Reflecting on the fact that our lives are composed of different levels, I can see that this is true for the universe as well. I enjoy visiting the American Museum of Natural History in Manhattan. My favorite place in the museum is the planetarium. I love learning about outer space, and the exhibits in this part of the museum really spark my imagination. The sheer quantity of galaxies and stars, along with the immense expansiveness of outer space, are mind-boggling. Just going outside on a clear night and gazing up at the stars, knowing that I could be looking at light from hundreds of years ago, captivates me.

To us humans, Earth is a huge blue-and-green planet that we call home. However, in the grand scheme of the universe, we are but a speck of dust. When I think about the amount of conflict and warring that occurs on this beautiful planet, with opposing sides being certain of the integrity and importance of their cause, it all seems so miniscule in the context of this vast universe. Viewing things from the greater perspective of the cosmos, it almost seems as if there should be no reason for so much strife.

Takeaways

- There are many potential levels of understanding in our lives and climbing these levels will enable us to grow as people. The best way to climb is to learn. How can we learn? Once again, by seeking the advice of others, reading an article or a book, or asking somebody who has done it before.
- When you find yourself in difficult situations or conflict, try to step away and see your circumstances from someplace outside yourself. You may very well gain a greater understanding and come up with a creative and practical solution.

CHAPTER 15

TEACHERS

In an earlier section, I mentioned the importance of teachers, stating that everything that occurs in life does so to impart a lesson. I have acquired this concept from several books and have appreciated it at work many times in my own life. My cancer diagnosis allowed me to open my eyes to my own eating habits and the dangers of processed foods. Mayra's absolute selflessness in caring for me when I was ill prompted me to take a closer look at myself and to emulate her great compassion. However, not until I really looked back on numerous events in my life did I fully realize the truth that everything happens for a reason.

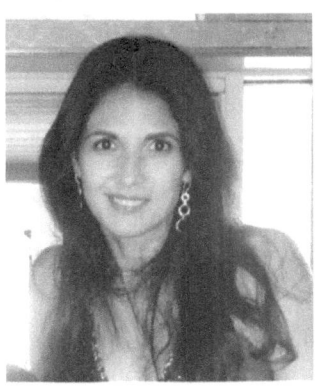

My #1 Teacher

I always considered myself to be a person of great patience. This was a quality of which I was proud. Moreover, I enjoyed this feeling of pride for many years. However, things seemed to have changed in December 2004. Early one morning during that month, after a mostly sleepless night, my life changed forever. It was the day Joshua was born. He was a true bundle of joy, a beautiful baby boy. I loved him the moment I laid eyes on him. However, as a first-time parent, I had absolutely no inkling of what I was in for.

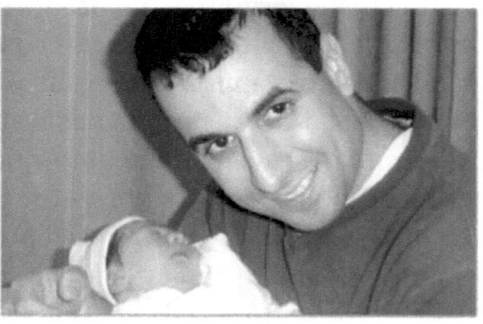

Josh's Birthday

Like all normal babies, Josh did not sleep through the night, and neither did we. I learned that babies require lots of attention during the day as well. I swiftly discovered that the free time I had previously cherished was disappearing. Activities such as reading, exercising, going to the store, and even going to the bathroom became huge challenges (it's difficult to relax on the toilet with a screaming newborn in the next room). Whatever patience I thought I had was nowhere to be found. Taking care of a baby required an entirely new level of composure. During the early weeks and months of Josh's life, he became my teacher. He was instructing me in the art of patience.

Besides needing to feed him, change his diapers, tend to his needs, and entertain him, Josh found other creative ways to instill the lesson of patience into my head. One evening while he was an infant, I was performing a routine diaper change. Run-of-the-mill baby poop, no problem. After all, I was an expert by that time. Josh was near the edge of the bed, the changing pad was in place, his legs were up, the dirty diaper was removed, the baby wipes were opened, and I was ready to go. But, apparently, Josh was not done. To my great dismay, Josh started pooping again. Right then and there while I held his legs in the air. Even more alarming was the fact that this was no solid poop. No, not this time. This poop was yellow, watery, and, I might add, copious. It was like an ocean wave as it ran over the changing pad, comforter, and, last but certainly not least—my belly. Wait, it gets a little bit better. To top it all off, I had no shirt on. So it was just warm, yellow, watery poop on my bare belly. This memory will forever be etched into my mind. For some reason, I do not remember the cleanup as well as the feeling of warm liquid poop on my skin. However, I am fairly certain that I called for reinforcements (Mayra) to help. When I look back on this harrowing experience, I always crack a smile. I also realize that it was a drill in patience.

As an infant and toddler, Josh was indisputably an excellent teacher who taught us more than just patience. He taught us that babies need a routine at bedtime and that they are not supposed to watch cartoons at 10:00 p.m. He taught us that a toddler should not be left alone with the cat because he might decide to grasp him by the tail and drag him across the floor. Luckily, we had a very tame cat that did nothing more than meow for help. He showed us that when you are carrying your toddler in a crowded department store, you should keep a bit of distance from other people, otherwise he might decide to reach out and grab an innocent woman's hair. Fortunately, she was quite understanding. He also made it clear that you should always keep a close eye on your little boy while in a grocery store, or else he might come up with the idea to run through the aisles screaming, "Help!"

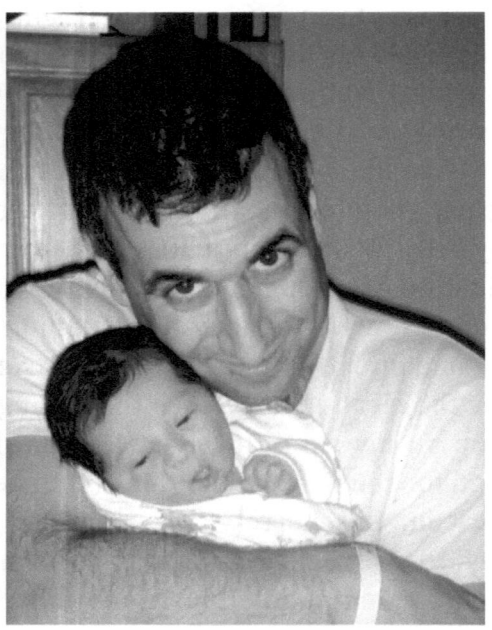

Joey's Birthday

When Joey was born two years later, we were a bit better off, as we had all the lessons Josh taught us under our belts. Although I did have more patience by then, Joey was quite eager to reinforce these lessons. As a toddler, there was one night when he would not stay in bed. He cried and climbed out of his crib. Not wanting him to walk around at night and get hurt, I got up and put him back in bed. A minute later, I heard him climbing out again and walking around his room. I got up and put him back in bed. A minute later, he did it again. And again. And again. And again. Shortly after his little game began, I decided to count the number of times he got out of bed. It was 110. That's right, he got out of bed—and I got up to put him back—110 times. Talk about a persistent kid.

Like Josh, Joey also enlightened us on many other subjects. He taught us that a two-year-old can climb out of a crib. He showed me that it can sometimes be dangerous to try to tickle a toddler, as I might get smacked in the face. We learned that a three-year-old can stand on a chair and help himself to some gum while his parents are not looking. He also showed me that little boys may have a warped sense of age when he said, "Daddy, you're forty-one. That's almost close to one hundred."

As Josh and Joey have gotten older, besides being two of my best friends, they continue to educate me. There have been times when I have gotten angry without basis, and they have called me out on it. They also continue to show me the importance of being childish and crazy at times. I still enjoy chasing them around the house and playing silly games such as "got you last." We wrestle and play-fight often. (Admittedly, it is much more of a challenge now than it was when they were smaller.) I look forward to having a life filled with jovial times and a continuing exchange of ideas with my two boys.

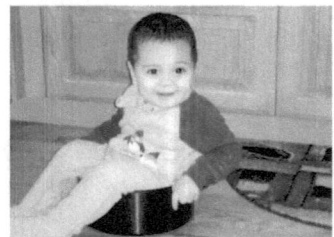
Joey getting comfy in a pot

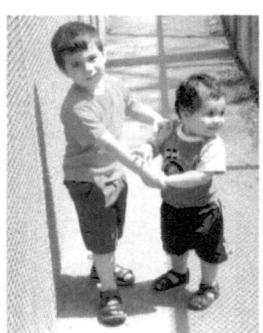
Going to the park

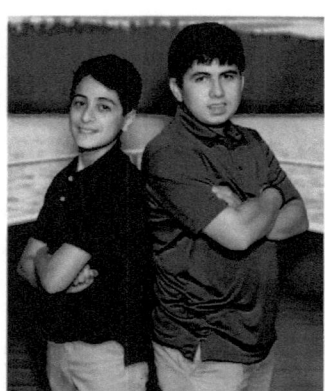
My handsome young men

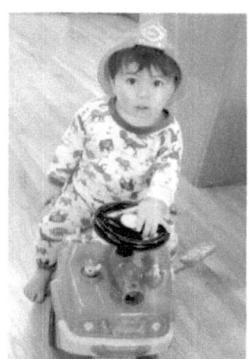
Josh and his firetruck

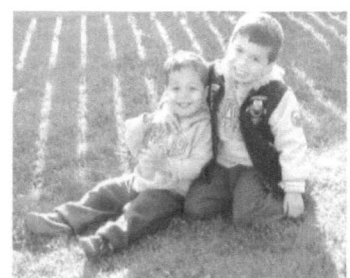
At the Fall Festival

Outside of family, I have learned things from many of my patients as well. There is one particular woman who stands out. Many years ago, I had the pleasure of meeting an older female. She was a spry senior citizen with a robust personality. She smiled a lot and was quite articulate. She demonstrated a wealth of knowledge on a wide range of topics. Among other things, I can remember her telling me, in great detail, how the ancient Romans built their roads. She was as sharp as a tack. She had just stopped driving a month prior due to poor eyesight. She recounted that, although she loved to drive, she openly accepted the loss of her driving privileges. She was very fond of one of the cars she used to drive, which happened to be a Corvette.

About a week before I met her, she had fallen and broken her arm and sustained an injury to her leg, which made it difficult for her to walk. She had her arm in a sling, and I could see bruising extending up to her collarbone. "No big deal," she had said. She was not only OK with this but also thriving in spite of it. She conveyed to me that she had always maintained an attitude of cheerfulness throughout her life. When life presented her with adversities, she responded with contentment. She believed it was the reason she had lived such a long and healthy life. When I asked her age, her answer astonished me. Ninety-five. Wow! I would never have guessed. As an emergency medicine physician, I come across quite a few nonagenarians. However, very rarely have I encountered one as lively and bubbly as my new friend. She taught me that her attitude toward life helped keep her healthy, intelligent, and exuberant.

It is obvious that I have had many wonderful teachers during my fifty years. It turns out, though, that I have found great teachers not only in humans but also in other creatures, specifically dogs and earthworms. Buddy, Rocky, and Bailey have taught me a great deal. First and foremost, they live in the present. Unlike humans, they do not appear to dwell on things that have already happened. If they do something naughty, such as stealing someone's dinner, they enjoy their bonus treat and seem to be done with it. By the same token, when they are reprimanded for their bad behavior, they hold no grudges. A moment later they are back to their usual playful selves. They also treasure their family, provide abundant amounts of love, and seek the same in return. When I'm gone for even a short time to run a quick errand, upon returning home they are excitedly wagging their tails, eager to greet me. When they are sick or injured, they don't complain. They may be a bit more calm than usual, but they will wag their tails, lick us, and still radiate happiness.

I did mention earthworms. That was not a typo. Earthworms can be great teachers. Have you ever walked outside after a heavy rainfall and noticed earthworms strewn across the asphalt? Sometimes there are so many of them that I find myself paying careful attention to every step, lest I create a massacre of worms. Occasionally I will pause and observe for a moment. I'll notice that while some are actively wriggling around, others are lying still. As I reflect on these little creatures, it seems to me that they may have different personalities. Although some seem to be quite motivated to get back to the soil in which they live, others appear to be fairly comfortable and indifferent with regard to their surroundings.

I remember one morning many years ago as I waited with my son at the school bus stop. The grass was muddy and there were puddles scattered about. As I looked down, I became intrigued by an earthworm a short distance away. This tiny organism seemed to be full of energy as it vigorously wiggled and twisted about, apparently trying to make its way back to the soil that it was evicted from by the prior night's rainfall. Its home lay a mere few inches away, perhaps a significant distance from a worm's perspective. As I watched my motivated companion, I leaned over to pick it up and placed it on the soil it longed for.

A short while later, it dawned on me. My earthworm friend inspired me to lend it a hand. The sheer desire that it demonstrated via its energy and perseverance moved me to help. I came to appreciate that what is true for earthworms is also true for us.

Takeaways

- Even if you believe that you are an expert on a subject, there may very well be more to learn.
- A good attitude will help you to live a good life.
- Be present.
- If you have a worthy objective in mind and display vitality and perseverance throughout the journey to achieve your goal, there will be others along the way who will help. Be diligent and honest in your efforts, and you will not be alone.

CHAPTER 16

A Backward Society?

In prior sections, I spent some time discussing the importance of perspective. I would like to discuss this topic once again. However, this time I would like to examine this concept as it relates to health. More specifically, I would like to share my thoughts and feelings regarding the way I see the current state of health care in our country. Although this may very well apply to other provinces around the globe, because I am not as familiar with medicine outside the United States, I will limit my discussion to the way I see it in this country.

I will start out by saying that I think we have everything backward. Please do not misunderstand. The lifesaving advances that have come about in medicine are nothing short of miraculous. I have cared for countless people who were rushed into the emergency department on an ambulance gurney, in critical condition and knocking on death's door. They all would have died if not for the expeditious treatment rendered. I've been involved in the treatment of innumerable patients in cardiac arrest with CPR in progress. Many of them lived to walk out of the hospital because of the medications and procedures given to them.

These are truly all wonderful advances that those in the field of medicine have enjoyed and that have benefited untold numbers of people. Nevertheless, I sincerely believe that we have everything *backward*. Why do I say this? I'll begin my response by sharing the information contained in many patients' medical records. The following is a typical example. As I click open the record on the computer, I will read the following:

Fifty-eight-year-old male with a medical history of DM, HTN, hyperlipidemia, CAD, CHF, GERD, and arthritis who presents to the emergency department with a complaint of chest pain ...

We use lots of acronyms in medicine. They certainly provide an efficient shorthand method of rapidly relaying information. The following will provide clarification:

> DM = diabetes mellitus
> HTN = hypertension (high blood pressure)
> CAD = coronary artery disease (blockages in the blood vessels of the heart)
> CHF = congestive heart failure
> GERD = gastroesophageal reflux disease (acid reflux)
> There are many more acronyms that those in the medical field commonly employ. A few additional examples include the following:
> COPD = chronic obstructive pulmonary disease (e.g., emphysema)
> CVA = cerebrovascular accident (stroke)
> MI = myocardial infarction (heart attack)
> PVD = peripheral vascular disease (blockages in blood vessels of the arms and legs)

ESRD = end-stage renal disease (renal failure, typically on dialysis)
RA = rheumatoid arthritis
SLE = systemic lupus erythematosus (lupus)
IBD = inflammatory bowel disease (Crohn's disease or ulcerative colitis)
PUD = peptic ulcer disease (ulcers in the stomach or intestines)
Hyperlipidemia = high cholesterol
Arthritis = joint pain

Returning to the record of our fifty-eight-year-old gentleman who came to the hospital for chest pain, I note that he is on multiple medications: two for diabetes, two for blood pressure, one for high cholesterol, a blood thinner for his CAD, a water pill for his CHF, an antacid medication for his GERD, and a pain medication for his arthritis. That's nine medications. Moreover, unless he makes some changes, I would bet money that his medication list is going to grow even more over the next several years.

Perusing a bit more of his record, I note that he has had a cardiac catheterization, with a stent placed in his heart.

Upon talking to this patient, he tells me that he has been having pressure-like chest pain since the morning. The pain radiates to his left arm, and he also has nausea. An EKG (electrical tracing of the heartbeats) reveals a few minor changes that were not present on a prior EKG. His blood work is normal. However, his symptoms are concerning enough that I admit him to the hospital for further evaluation. While in the hospital, he will have more blood work done and will also likely have an echocardiogram (sonogram of the heart) to assess how well his heart is pumping. Depending on the results of his evaluation, he may be discharged to have a stress test, or he may need another cardiac catheterization to determine whether there are additional blockages in the blood vessels of his heart.

As I alluded to earlier, my fifty-eight-year-old patient is a representative example of the patients who come through the doors of the emergency department. Their medical records are filled with acronyms—CAD, CHF, HTN, COPD, CVA, DM, PVD, ESRD, and GERD, among others. Although I am not aware of acronyms for many types of cancer, it is also commonly found in many patients' medical histories, as is obesity. Typical medication lists contain at least five, and more often ten or greater, different prescriptions.

Many have had multiple life- and limb-saving procedures. CABG (coronary artery bypass graft) is a common one. This is basically a surgery wherein they remove veins from a limb and use them to "bypass" the diseased blood vessels of the heart. There are also bypass surgeries for the limbs, where a synthetic graft is used to divert blood flow around a diseased vessel and restore circulation to muscles and nerves. Many people suffering from strokes have been administered clot-busting medications, or they sometimes even have had the arteries of their brain cleared by specialized devices used to physically remove obstructing clots.

I see these conditions, medications, and procedures listed on so many patient charts that it has become commonplace. Everybody seems to have DM, HTN, high cholesterol, and CAD. It's just routine. So many people are on a slew of medications. Again, this seems typical. It's just the way things are—it has become normal to have multiple medical problems and to be on a variety of medications. Your chest pain may be the symptom of a heart attack. No worries. We can diagnose and fix that. You can have a cardiac catheterization and we'll open up the blocked artery with a stent. We will then start you on a few medications to keep things in check. Not a problem. You have just been diagnosed with high blood pressure or diabetes. That's a piece of cake (no pun intended). Here are a couple of prescriptions. They'll help you feel better. The health-care system has got you covered. In my humble opinion, this is *backward*.

Let me say it once again—modern medicine can do wonders. It can, and does, save lives. In addition, the men and women who work in healthcare are diligent and conscientious heroes, and I am fortunate to be part of a team of wonderful and caring people. But where does the ultimate responsibility for a person's health rest? Is it with medical practitioners and hospitals? *Most. Definitely. Not.* In my opinion, it is the person themselves who should be accountable for their own well-being. Caveat: Many of the disease conditions mentioned previously (known as chronic degenerative diseases) are often due to poor lifestyle choices and are largely preventable. However, when things have reached a critical point, complications are likely to occur that will require immediate care. Moreover, there are diseases out there that are not due to poor lifestyles. In addition, there will be occasions when disease processes, including the ones mentioned earlier, will occur even if you do take good care of yourself. *Thus, if you are feeling very ill, please seek urgent medical care.*

I feel that I see things differently from others. Regarding our health, I believe that there are two main paths from which we can choose. The first path has us eating poorly, being sedentary, developing one or more of these chronic degenerative diseases, and then being placed on medications and undergoing medical procedures. The second path has us eating well, moving our bodies regularly, and feeling wonderful. There will likely be no prescription medications or medical procedures on this path.

Should we be abusing the miraculous gift that is our body and just patching it up with bandages and controlling diseases with drugs? With the ever-increasing number of pharmaceuticals and medical technologies that are being developed, it can be easy to slowly destroy our bodies and then give the medical establishment the responsibility to fix us. Our focus should not be on figuring out what doctors can do to save us after we have mistreated ourselves for so many years. Instead, our attention should be on cherishing the gift we have been given and treating it like the treasure it is. The choice is ours.

How do you see your life in the present? How about the future you? Your body will only be able to withstand poor treatment for a finite amount of time before it starts breaking down. I just don't see how it makes sense to spend years eating poorly and then getting ourselves placed on a laundry list of medications to help our body regulate the disease states that many times *we have created. Why take medications and eat bad foods at the same time?* In my opinion, this is absurd. I submit that it is a much better idea to provide our body with the nutrients it craves and the regular exercise it needs. This will significantly decrease the risk of developing these chronic degenerative diseases and being saddled with the medication list that goes along with them.

Regarding medications, a fact that is worth noting is the presence of side effects. Medications come with many side effects, some more than others. A few common reactions are nausea, vomiting, low blood pressure, dizziness, falls, bleeding, constipation, infection, liver damage, kidney damage, and abnormal heart rhythms. Moreover, side effects are not the only concern. Medications can interact with each other and generate an entirely new set of side effects. Overall, the unintended consequences of medication use, which are called adverse drug reactions, are a serious consideration. Studies have shown that 3 to 7 percent of all hospitalizations are the result of these reactions. These reactions were also found to be the fourth to sixth leading causes of death in hospitalized patients in the United States.[1]

I would like to switch gears and spend a moment discussing another facet of modern medicine—procedures. Specifically, I'd like to focus on cardiac catheterizations. Again, the available technology and ability of medical practitioners to offer these treatments to people are truly miraculous, and they do save lives. It happens every day. A person comes into the emergency department looking ill, dripping with sweat, and complaining of chest pain because they are having a heart attack. It is a truly remarkable thing to have a team of nurses, doctors, and other hospital staff come together, administer lifesaving medications, and have that patient whisked off to the cardiac catheterization lab where they will likely get a stent to open up a blocked blood vessel. Typically, the time when the patient walks through the door of the emergency department to the time they head to the catheterization lab is thirty minutes or less. Amazing. This person now has a new lease on life.

My big question is whether the heart attack had to happen in the first place. If the person just described (perhaps it could be you) cared for their body and gave it what it needed, they might not have required an emergency, lifesaving medical procedure in the first place. Is it really the cardiologist who is ultimately responsible for your health—*or is it you?*

In an earlier chapter, I told the story of how shocked I was when I could not save a young woman whose cause of death ended up being a heart attack. Furthermore, over the years, I have treated countless people who sought care for complications of one or more lifestyle-related diseases. Regrettably, these people had been slowly destroying their bodies as a result of poor nutrition and unhealthy choices. I recall taking care of a forty-eight-year-old male who came in for a minor complaint. However, it turned out that, the week before, he had been hospitalized for a heart attack requiring a cardiac catheterization and a stent placement. Then there was a forty-year-old male who came to the hospital because of a urinary infection. I was surprised to note in his medical record that he had had a heart attack seven years earlier—at the ripe old age of thirty-three.

These unfortunate realities genuinely sadden me. I feel so horrible knowing that people are literally slowly killing themselves. Moreover, these maladies are not just affecting adults. Our children are developing these conditions as well. Prior to a few years ago, I never would have thought that children could have high cholesterol. I was thus astonished to learn that, in 2009, 2.8 million prescriptions for cholesterol-lowering drugs were written by pediatricians.[2] That is just insane, for lack of a better word.

According to the Centers for Disease Control and Prevention, 7 percent of children and adolescents ages six to nineteen have elevated cholesterol levels.[3] Even more frightening were the results of a study that was conducted in Louisiana. This study looked at young people and found the existence of plaque in the coronary arteries (blood vessels supplying blood to the heart). Plaque comprises deposits of fat and other substances that form within your blood vessels. It is these deposits that can lead to vascular disease, heart attacks, and strokes. In this study, plaque was found in children as young as age two, all the way up to adults aged thirty-nine, with the prevalence of the plaque increasing in the older age groups.[4] Again, for lack of a better word, that is just insane. Think about it for a moment. Vigorous and happy two-year-olds are starting to develop heart disease. Furthermore, youngsters are also developing type 2 diabetes. This is a condition that in the past was rarely seen in children. It is now becoming a more frequent problem in adolescents and preteens, some as young as ten years old.[5]

Again, although it is important to know the facts, I do not feel that I need them to prove to myself that the state of health in this country is appalling. I say this because I can see people's health declining every time I go to work. I have already spoken about many of the adult patients I treat. As far as children are concerned, I have cared for so many youngsters (adolescents, preteens, and even younger children) who are obese. I have treated teens who already take medications because they have developed adult-onset diabetes. Gallstones, which is a condition I used to see only in adults, is becoming a condition of adolescents as well. Granted, I work in only a single hospital. However, by reading and listening to others, I have learned that this health crisis is unquestionably not isolated to my small part of the country.

Notice that I said *health crisis* as opposed to *health-care crisis*. This is not a disaster of the health-care system and the medical establishment. This is a catastrophe that we have brought on ourselves. How so? The answer to this question, once again, can be found in our lifestyles. Many of us consume diets containing an abundance of processed foods and severely lacking in colorful fruits and vegetables. Countless numbers of people live a sedentary lifestyle. We have *chosen* to do this to ourselves.

I realize that I have probably disclosed many frightening facts. My intention regarding this health-related discussion thus far has not been to alarm you. My main objective has been to generate awareness. I understand that a large number of people living unhealthy lifestyles may be oblivious to this fact. They may be unaware that many of the processed foods they consume are slowly harming them. If you recall, I was one of those people. My goal is that everyone who reads this and who has not been taking care of themselves will appreciate the reality that they are likely going to fall ill. We can be better. It is never too late to change.

My humble opinion is that we need a paradigm shift. We should start doing things correctly right from the outset rather than living an unhealthy lifestyle and having things spiral out of control to the point where we all become medical statistics. Can we really do this? I believe that the answer is a resounding yes! I truly feel that all of us damaging our treasured bodies with poor nutrition and lack of movement can change the way we live. I would have no way of knowing exact numbers, but living a healthier life is something that thousands, perhaps millions, have already done. As I discussed earlier in this book, it's all about making good choices and taking action. It really is that simple.

Remember, it is what we do most of the time that counts. What do you need to do most of the time in order to live a healthier life? Refrain from or significantly decrease your intake of processed foods. Consume an abundance of colorful fruits and vegetables. Exercise on a regular basis. If you smoke or consume excessive amounts of alcohol, you should gradually decrease your usage and then stop completely. If you are already on medications for lifestyle-related diseases, there is a good chance that you will be able to reduce your intake or stop them altogether. Caveat number one: If you are under the care of a doctor, make these lifestyle changes, especially while beginning an exercise program, under their guidance. Caveat number two: Never stop taking prescription medications without your doctor's direction. Caveat number three: Alcohol withdrawal can be a life-threatening condition. If you are a longtime everyday drinker, you should not stop drinking abruptly unless under a doctor's guidance.

In the previous paragraph, I mentioned that you may be able to reduce or stop taking prescription medications if you adopt a healthier lifestyle. This is because if you change the way you live, eat, and move, then the progression of many of these chronic diseases can be slowed or actually reversed. Yes—reversed! This even includes coronary artery disease (blocked blood vessels in the heart).[6] This is not only an amazing fact but also can provide hope and inspiration for countless people.

Some people might be concerned because of their family's health history. Perhaps both of their parents suffered heart attacks at relatively young ages. Or maybe there is a strong family history of diabetes or cancer. Do not fret. There is more good news. You are not doomed to suffer solely because of your heredity. Science has found that your genes are not definitive determinants of your destiny. A field of science called epigenetics has shown us this. What we have learned is that there are certain parts of the body's DNA (genetic material) that act like switches, enabling many genes to either be turned on or off. For example, let's say that a person has many close family members who suffered heart attacks at a young age. In this case, it certainly does seem as though there is a strong genetic propensity toward the development of heart disease. However, often the "heart disease" gene needs to be turned on for the damage to begin. Thus, if you have this gene and you eat a horrible diet and are mostly sedentary, there is a good chance that this gene will be activated. Conversely, if you eat a healthy diet, exercise regularly, and are a mostly calm person, then the chance that your "heart disease" gene will be activated, leading to the development of a heart attack, will be significantly diminished. This, again, is wonderful news for all.[7,8]

So what do you think? Would you like to help create that new paradigm I mentioned earlier? Would you like to cease doing things backward? Would you like to stop eating poorly and consequently traveling down the path of illness and a life filled with prescription drugs and medical procedures? Would you instead like to become an *active* participant in the evolution of a healthier you? Of a healthier population? If so, please read on. I applaud you. Each one of us can make changes that will get the ball rolling. If you are already health conscious—kudos! If not, don't worry. As you have learned, many times these horrendous chronic diseases are not only preventable but also *reversible.* It's up to you to decide which path you are going to take. (Cancer is one lifestyle-related disease that is not likely to be reversible with lifestyle modifications alone. Care by a medical specialist is required for treatment.)

Before we continue our journey, I would like to take a little time to ensure that we have the proper perspective on things. First off—making changes of this magnitude should in no way be a chore. Identifying a healthy lifestyle as an obligation will not be fun. It will also set you up for failure. Everything that you do to take care of yourself should give you pleasure. Eating nutritious foods is critical. However, if you don't like what you are eating, you will not last long. That being said, there are an abundance of ways to prepare and eat fresh fruits, vegetables, nuts, grains, beans, and seeds in delicious and healthy ways. Another important point to recognize is that it may take several exposures to a new food to develop a taste for it. If you are currently a big fan of processed, sweet, and fatty foods, you should not view a healthy change in diet as having to rid your pantry of foods that you like but rather as *gaining* the opportunities to add other types of mouthwatering cuisine to your life.

Besides finding wholesome foods that you love, there is an additional salient point that you should appreciate about nutritious foods. The healthy foods that I mentioned earlier—fresh fruits, vegetables, nuts, grains, beans, and seeds—are packed with an array of vitamins, minerals, antioxidants, and phytochemicals. These nutrients are essential for combating disease and maintaining good health. Moreover, the greater variety in the colors of the fruits and vegetables you eat will provide you with a greater diversity of nutrients. When it comes to being healthy, these substances are natural—and superior—options to prescription medications. Actually, most prescription medications don't really make you healthy; they just help control the symptoms of diseases that often *you* created. Natural, unprocessed foods are truly the best medicines. What do you think about letting food be your medicine? (To reiterate, never stop taking prescription medications without your health-care provider's guidance). An additional important note that I would like to make is that prescription drugs are not evil. There are many pharmaceuticals that are lifesaving and have enabled people afflicted with numerous conditions to live happy lives. My concern is when people use medications to treat the symptoms of diseases that developed because of poor lifestyle choices.

After reading this, some people may feel that it is too difficult to eat healthy foods most of the time, for a couple of reasons. First, they may assume that the cost of wholesome, unprocessed foods is prohibitive. This is a valid concern, and I decided to do some research on the topic. I went online and searched for samples of both wholesome, fresh foods as well as processed foods. I recorded the prices for each food and calculated the cost for its suggested serving size. I then compiled a list comparing options for both categories of food, along with their cost per serving, in a sample menu for a day. Here's what it looks like:

	Natural Foods (cost per serving)	Processed Foods (cost per serving)
Breakfast	Rolled oats (~26¢)	Typical boxed cereal (~26¢)
Snack	Banana (~23¢) Nuts (~70¢) Apple (~50¢) Grapes (~24¢) Baby carrots (~20¢) Hummus (~47¢)	Candy bar (~70¢) Chocolate chip granola bar (~25¢) Chocolate chip cookies (~18¢ per 3 cookies)

		Chocolate cupcake (~35¢) Potato chips (~25¢)
Lunch	Salad with mixed greens, tomatoes, almonds, red onions, and balsamic dressing (~$4.85)	Quarter-pound burger with cheese and french fries (~$5.79)
Dinner	Quinoa with beans and two vegetables (~$2.46)	Sirloin steak and boxed mashed potatoes (~$2.83) Frozen dinner of pasta and cheese (~$1.98)

As you can see, the prices of natural, healthy foods are often equivalent to, and sometimes even less expensive than, processed foods. Thus, if cost is a concern, this information should help allay some worries. In addition, buying store-brand items and purchasing larger-size quantities will also help lower the costs. People may also be hesitant regarding the time factor. I realize that many of us are quite busy, myself included. Between work and family obligations, it may seem impossible to spend a few hours cooking a decent, healthy meal. I believe that the solution to this problem is proper planning. On the days when you are off from work, plan out your meals, especially your dinner menu, for the next few days or week. Make a trip to the grocery store and buy what you need. Then spend some time prepping and perhaps even preparing some of the items needed for your meals. You will then be set with healthy meals for at least a few days. I am confident that investing this time once or twice a week will pay great dividends for you. If there are children in your home, let them be involved as well. This will help them come to appreciate the joys of preparing real, natural foods that can be enjoyed together.

The same fundamental truth regarding enjoying the food you eat also applies to movement. Moving your body on a regular basis is, without a doubt, a health-promoting activity. This, too, should not be viewed as a chore. Granted, giving yourself the regular exercise that you need is likely going to require more effort than eating healthily. Nonetheless, this should not be thought of as a duty. After all, this type of work can be a lot of fun. Getting your heart rate up, building up a sweat, and feeling pumped release your body's natural endorphins (feel-good chemicals) and many times provide you with a natural high. You *will* enjoy this. Physical exercise also enables you to become more focused and to think more clearly. I know there are a multitude of scientific studies that demonstrate this relationship. However, I can attest to these benefits from personal experience.

Takeaways

- Unfortunately, chronic diseases have become the norm.
- Lifesaving miracles can be performed by practitioners of modern medicine. No question there. The true question is whether you should allow the state of your health to deteriorate to the point where it is in need of such intervention.

- These frightening health issues affect children as well.
- A paradigm shift is necessary.
- Many times, chronic diseases can be prevented and even reversed.
- Your genes do not dictate your future.
- You have the power to change the path of your life and your health.
- Eat nutrient-packed natural food and move your body. Be consistent with both.
- Eating healthy foods does not have to be significantly more expensive or time consuming than eating unhealthy foods.

CHAPTER 17

CLEAR GOALS AND CONSISTENT ACTION

OK—let's dive in. Remember, if you have a long path ahead on your journey to good health, enjoy it every step of the way. Sometimes it's difficult to figure out where to start. If that's the case, don't worry. The first thing you need to do is to determine where you are now and where you want to go. As it relates to health, what does your life look like? What foods do you eat every day? How much physical activity do you get? Pay close attention to these things over the course of a few days to a week and record your observations. Regarding foods—how many meals and snacks do you eat each day? What kinds of foods do you feed yourself, and what are your portion sizes? Be honest with yourself. Concerning exercise—how much activity are you giving yourself? What types of activity do you participate in, how often, and for how long? Again, be truthful. You deserve it. Don't worry if your current situation seems discouraging. You are taking this important step to create a better version of yourself. Thus, it's important to have a clear starting point. You'll see. Take your time and do this well. You can pause here for a few days if you like. I promise, I will still be here when you return.

Now that you have a clear picture of where you are, it is time to create a picture of equal, if not greater, clarity of where you want to go. You must decide how you want your life to be in the coming months and years. You have to visualize your life at a specific time in the future. Notice that I said *specific*. When setting goals, it is essential to be specific. Develop goals, and then pick a particular date on which each goal should be accomplished. For example, suppose you have a goal to lose twenty pounds. You might decide that, in nine months, on June 12, you will have met your goal. Maybe your goal is to be able to jog two miles. Give yourself a set date—perhaps August 1—to achieve this.

As I have just alluded to, it is also important to be specific about the goals themselves. Vagueness will not work well here. "I want to lose a few pounds soon" is not a good goal. "I want to lose two pounds by the last day of the month" is much more effective. "I want to add more fruits and vegetables into my diet" is a weak motivator. However, stating, "Within two weeks I will have added two servings of fruits and a serving of vegetables into my daily diet" will really get you moving.

Aside from specificity, another important factor is to write down your goals. The physical act of writing them down makes them more real. I feel that this also creates some accountability. However, don't just record them in a place where you will never see them again. You've heard the expression—out of sight, out of mind. You don't want this to be the case for your aspirations. Write them on sticky notes and place them in visible locations where you are going to see them several times throughout the day. Suggestions include the bathroom mirror, the refrigerator, the kitchen cabinet, your desk at the office, your wallet or purse, and your cell phone.

When establishing goals, make sure that they are reasonable. Asking yourself to do something that is going to be very difficult will likely be a setup for failure. For instance, if you are currently at an unhealthy place in your life, then setting a goal to lose fifty pounds and being able to run five miles in three months is probably not going to work out too well. That is not to say that you can't have huge aspirations for yourself. Big dreams are awesome! However, the better way to begin is to break your colossal goal into many smaller goals, each with its own completion date. Focus on the smaller goals. This will allow you to see each individual goal as attainable and prevent you from becoming overwhelmed. You will also get to celebrate multiple victories along the way. Thus, a much better way of expressing the earlier goal would be to say that you are going to lose two pounds in the next thirty days and jog a quarter mile within the next two months. These small and more easily achievable goals can be repeated over and over. Not overwhelming in the least. However, at the end of two years, you will be fifty pounds lighter and be jogging five miles.

Thus far, we have created clear pictures of where we are and where we wish to be. We have been specific and written our goals down in places where we will see them several times each day. We have broken large goals into smaller, more manageable ones. Fantastic! In addition, always remember our friend—momentum. As we move forward, momentum will develop and keep us going. Things will start to get easier. We will be in the zone. We can do this. We will become unstoppable!

Now that everything has been set up, it is time to take action. Not just any old action, but *consistent* action. A good place to begin is to look at your daily habits. What types of foods do you like, and how much of them do you eat? How much physical activity are you getting? Start small and begin making little adjustments in the form of one or two small changes every several days. If you currently enjoy a pastry every night, then how about enjoying an apple every other night instead? If you eat a fried, high-fat dinner a few times each week, how about eating a meal that is filled with vegetables and lighter on the fat on one of those nights? Take baby steps and slowly advance. *Watch your portion sizes.* Remember to try to eat foods that are unprocessed and as close to the earth as possible. Slowly cut out sweets, fats, and sugary drinks. Need recipe ideas? Perfect—ideas are great. There is an abundance of both free and purchasable recipes that are available in books, through phone apps, and on the internet.

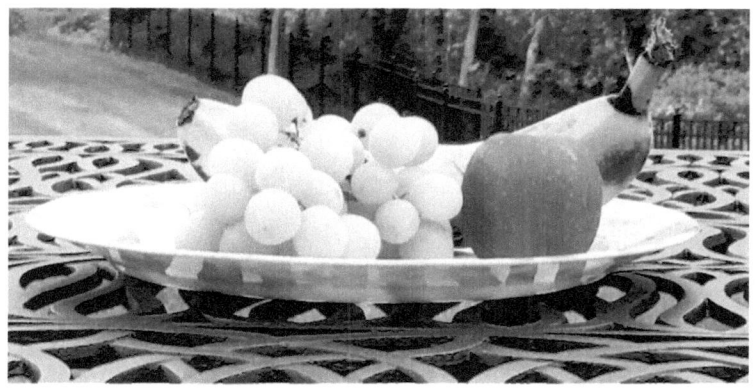

Some delicious and healthy snacks

If you are in the habit of being sedentary, the time has come to break that habit and replace it with the habit of physical activity. Moreover, when it comes to physical activity, just like food, find things that you enjoy. I would not want you to be jogging five miles each day if you loathe jogging. You'll be miserable. Although, many times after performing an activity awhile, you start to get into a groove and develop an affinity for it. You might just learn that you really enjoy something that you previously thought you hated. There are a multitude of activities to try—everything from organized sports to running, hiking, martial arts, bicycling, dancing, and so many more. Remember, take small steps. Find something that you love, get out there, and have fun!

Enjoying your healthy lifestyle with someone else can be terrific. Having a buddy is wonderful. If you have a friend, coworker, or family member who also has the goal of developing a healthier lifestyle, ask if they would like to take this journey with you. Perhaps more than one person would be interested. You can be accountable to each other, motivate one another, and feed off each other's energy. Even if there is nobody in your immediate network who shares your health goals, perhaps there is someone you trust with whom you can share your aspirations. This person can be a motivator as well as someone who holds you accountable for the actions you have committed to taking. After all, if you feel as though you are too busy, it is much easier to keep the fact that you are planning to skip your workout to yourself rather than tell someone who is going to hold you accountable for your actions (or inactions).

My son Joey has turned into a fantastic partner. Although both Josh and Joey are disciplined when it comes to schoolwork, Joey has also developed great discipline when it comes to exercise. He works out six days each week—Sunday through Friday. Saturday is his rest day. He bench presses twice per week, works out his arms three times per week, and works out his legs three times per week. He works on his abs all six days. This is his exercise schedule, and he sticks to it. No excuses. It turns out that he motivated Josh to join him in his workouts every day. He inspires and pushes Josh to keep exercising hard in order to become stronger and healthier, and Josh has shown great progress since he became his brother's workout buddy.

Regarding exercise, even with buddies or partners, there are going to be times when you just don't feel like working out. You're too tired. It's raining outside. You don't feel like driving to the gym. You are just not in the mood. These can be tough times. This is when you must summon your inner strength and just get moving. Start slowly. If you're running, just take one step at a time. If you're lifting weights, focus only on the next rep. Earlier, I told you the story of the day I went running when I just did not feel like it. I ended up having a great run. That was not the only day I was not in the mood to exercise. There have been many others. For whatever reason, I often have outstanding workouts on those days when I just didn't feel like moving. I know that my great friend momentum helps me tremendously.

I frequently have this experience after a night shift. As an ER doctor, I work several nights each month. If I am working two consecutive nights, then after the second night, I will often run or ride my bike after I get home in the morning. Let me tell you, it is not easy. On my way home, I feel so tired after having run around the emergency department for twelve hours. All I can think about is my bed. However, if I say that I am going to run, then I am going to run. The first ten or fifteen minutes are usually quite demanding. However, after that, it starts to get progressively easier. I typically end up having great runs after my night shifts. Moreover, I am not the only one who does this. Several of my coworkers do the same thing after working a night shift. I applaud all those who accept and conquer this challenge.

Another helpful piece of advice, especially when starting out, is to keep a written record of your progress. This could be in a journal, on a calendar, or on your phone or computer. Having a visual record of your progress is tremendously helpful. Being able to view your efforts and accomplishments in a physical form serves as a motivational tool and helps you build momentum.

Many years ago, Mayra had fallen into a slump of sorts. She had always been disciplined about exercising regularly. Then a time came when she lost her motivation and stopped working out. Although she was upset about this, she couldn't seem to get moving again. In trying to figure out a way to help her, I had the idea to give her a special gift. I purchased a twelve-month schedule book, and on the last page, I wrote exercise goals for a month, along with a grading scale. For example, four workouts per month would earn her a grade of "You've taken a big step in the right direction. Keep going!"; eight workouts per month would earn her a grade of "Nicely done!"; twelve workouts per month would earn her a grade of "You're on fire!"; and fifteen workouts per month would earn her a grade of "Outstanding!"

She started to exercise and use the calendar, marking off the days that she worked out. After a few weeks, she had developed a great deal of momentum and kept going strong. She loved it and felt great. She became unstoppable. Just as it was for Mayra, an exercise calendar can be a powerful tool on your health journey.

I would like to reinforce a topic that I mentioned earlier—failure. Failures are important and are often critical for growth in all aspects of life. It is important to view failures as teachers and not as reasons to become discouraged and self-critical. We must fail, gain something from our failure, and then move forward. I would posit that the same applies if you are trying to attain health and fitness goals. There are likely going to be times when you fall short of your goals. Perhaps you were aiming to lose three pounds by the end of the month and you lost only one. Maybe you wanted to be able to jog a mile in two months and you haven't quite gotten there despite being consistent. These apparent failures may very well happen. But don't despair; this is OK. It's also often a necessary part of the road to success.

We are human and thus fallible. There are going to be times when we fail to meet our established goals. It happens to everyone, and it does not make you any less of a person. I realize that it is quite easy for me to make this statement as I am sitting here typing. However, that does not negate its truth. As you have learned, I have experienced many failures in life. Sure, when it happens, I feel disappointed in myself for a bit. This is a normal emotional reaction to defeat, and you should surely allow yourself to experience it. But then it is time to move on. Furthermore, as with all failures, you might just learn something and find a better approach.

Takeaways

- Where are you now, and where do you want to be?
- Create specific and reasonable goals and write them down.
- Take consistent action.
- Eat healthy food and engage in activities that you enjoy.
- Get a buddy.
- There will be days when you just don't feel like it. Do it anyway.

- Keep a calendar.
- Failures will occur. Learn from them if possible and then move on.

CHAPTER 18

YOU ARE UNIQUE

As you proceed on the path to becoming a healthier person, it is a great idea to have aspirations. Maybe you want to lose a predetermined amount of weight. Perhaps you want six-pack abs. These desires will help propel you forward. You may decide to use pictures of athletes as motivation. Again, this is a good thing. Having a visual depiction of where you want to end up can be powerful. However, I would like to offer a word of advice. You are your own person. You are so very special in your own right. You are unique, and there is nobody else on this planet of nearly *eight billion* people who is exactly like you. Pretty impressive, isn't it?

My point is that you are not, and should not aim to look exactly like, someone else. You are not them—*you are you.* You can, by all means, use other people as motivators on your quest to be healthier. Actually, you can use other people as motivators for pretty much any goal you set for yourself. Moreover, you can unquestionably learn from others. Nevertheless, always remember that you are unique. The only person you should be competing with is yourself. Nobody else. Rather than trying to exactly mimic another person's level of fitness or success, you should focus on trying to make *yourself* a little bit better every single day.

To emphasize, your focus should be gradual self-improvement. However, there may be days when you become frustrated. Remember, we are imperfect by nature. It may feel as though you are losing your motivation. You may question yourself as to whether it is worth all the effort. When these moments occur, I urge you to think about the future you; consider your choices and ask yourself *rather* questions. For example, would you rather eat and enjoy lots of unhealthy processed and junk foods on a regular basis and significantly increase the *very real risk* that you will later go on to develop obesity, diabetes, high blood pressure, heart disease, and cancer? Or would you rather eat and *enjoy* flavorful natural foods on a regular basis, knowing that they will help keep you healthy, energetic, and focused? Would you rather lounge on the sofa watching television for several hours each day and become a less energetic person with poor focus? Or would you rather spend some of that time being physically active, remarkably raising the likelihood that your future you will remain vibrant and full of life?

I would like to remind you of the supreme importance of consistency. It is what you do most of the time that counts. Live a healthy lifestyle most of the time, and it is likely that you will enjoy vibrancy and good health. Live an unhealthy lifestyle most of the time, and it is likely that you will suffer the devastating effects of multiple chronic diseases. Having said that, it is perfectly fine to indulge on occasion. If you crave pizza, ice cream, or chocolate mousse, it's all right to enjoy these foods. Once again, it's what you do most of the time that counts. Remember, just as eating a single fruit salad is not going to make you healthy, eating a single piece of chocolate cake is not going to give you diabetes. Be consistent in eating healthier foods, and you will be fine.

Takeaways

- Use others for motivation.
- Compete only with yourself.
- Always think about the future you.
- It is what you do most of the time that counts.

CHAPTER 19

FINAL THOUGHTS

It is my sincere wish that my experiences and thoughts thus far in my life will benefit you in yours. I would like to share three final lessons with you. The first one relates to belief. I trust in the power of belief. My opinion is that if a person truly has faith that they will accomplish something good and worthwhile, then their desire will become reality. This, of course, will not just happen spontaneously. It will require the necessary planning, practice, and effort. The story of Roger Bannister is a perfect illustration of this idea. Mr. Bannister was a runner. You see, for all the time that track and field records had been kept, nobody had ever run a mile in four minutes. In fact, it was deemed impossible by many for a human to run so fast for such a distance. It was a barrier that no person could break. That was, until May 6, 1954, arrived. Roger Bannister had resolved to be the first person to run a mile in four minutes. On that day, he ran a mile in three minutes and fifty-nine seconds. He broke through barriers that had never been breached.

This story is incredible by itself. However, the truly amazing part of this story is that his record lasted only forty-six days. Within the next year, another three runners broke the four-minute barrier. Moreover, since that time, well over a thousand runners have also broken the four-minute-mile record. How could it be that nobody could run a four-minute mile prior to 1954 and then all of a sudden four people can do it within a year, with greater than a thousand more to follow over the ensuing decades? The answer lies in the fact that the barrier was not physical but mental. It existed only in the minds of runners. As soon as Roger Bannister proved that it could be done, the barrier was broken.

This story serves as proof that many times our own barriers do not exist outside us but rather within us. Never give up on your worthwhile dreams.

This takes me to the second lesson that I would like to impart. Although belief is important, its power cannot be realized without the proper attitude and mindset. I have learned this not only from my ninety-five-year-old friend but also from my own daily life. I'm sure that many of you have had the same commonplace experiences that I am about to share. There are some days when I get up on the wrong side of the bed. I don't give my wife a smile or a good-morning kiss. She senses something amiss and distances herself. I will be impatient with my boys. As my morning progresses, I can't seem to find papers that I was planning to work on. I might try to do some work online and discover that the computer has frozen. Other small things seem to go wrong over the course of the day.

Conversely, life seems much easier when I am in a good mood. When I choose to have feelings of gratitude and cheerfulness toward those around me, my day is quite pleasant. I wake up with a smile and take a moment to make coffee for my wife. She smiles and hugs me. My boys laugh with me. Whatever tasks I have planned usually go well. Moreover, even if they don't, I have already chosen to be happy and thankful, so it's OK either way.

I learned that the expression *what goes around comes around* really is true. Hostility begets hostility. Kindness begets kindness. Love begets love. Add value unto others and you will receive it in return. What we send out into the world will come back to us.

The last, but certainly not least, important lesson is gratitude. Be grateful. Believe me, I know that it can be difficult at times. But if you are breathing, then you have something to be thankful for.

Several years ago, one morning in July, we were leaving from New York to visit my sister in Virginia. That also happened to be the morning I woke up with lower back pain. I had never had back pain before, and I had not done anything the day prior to injure myself. I figured that it was probably some muscle stiffness that would resolve within a few hours. To my dismay, the pain decided not to resolve but instead continued to evolve. Two days later, I was experiencing pain in my right buttock that radiated down my right thigh. It was an intense, deep ache. I also had numbness in my ankle. It frequently hurt more to walk, and I sometimes could not find a comfortable position in which to sit or lie down. I chalked it up to sciatica that would last a week and then go away. Didn't happen. Five weeks later, I was walking around Disney World with the same deep ache in my leg.

Throughout much of this, I tried to practice something that I had learned many times over. The idea that what one focuses on grows stronger is a profound truth. Rather than focus on the pain, I would try to home in on the things I was grateful for. I would center my thoughts on the people I was with and the activities I was engaged in. I would think about the fact that I was so fortunate to be alive, healthy, and with my family. As I mentioned, this was not always easy to do. Nevertheless, when I was able to keep my thoughts focused on all the good in my life, I usually would not have pain. Moreover, if I did have pain, it would not bother me as much.

Focus on the good attributes in your life and be thankful. You will empower them to grow stronger.

I would like to end with a blog post that I wrote several years ago. I feel that it provides a rather good perspective on becoming your best self.

Early this summer I started my vegetable garden. I pulled up the weeds that had grown in the spring and put in fresh soil.

I planted a few different vegetables, including tomatoes. I had purchased them as small plants. They seemed so small and delicate—no more than six inches tall. Over the ensuing weeks, I tended to them regularly. I ensured that they were adequately watered and secured them to posts to assure they would be well supported.

Yesterday, as I admired the garden, something struck a chord within. I noticed just how much my tomato plants had grown. I had recognized this every time I cared for the garden. But yesterday I really *understood* it. They are at least two feet tall—very green and lush. They are so big that their leaves are overhanging the wooden planters. I even saw a small tomato here and there. They are truly majestic.

As I marveled at my garden, a concept came to mind: the plants are *supposed* to grow. I know it sounds obvious, but bear with me. The young seedlings were *meant* to develop and flourish. All that potential was in the tiny seeds from which they originated. They were destined to become magnificent wonders of nature.

The same is true for all creatures. Every living thing on this planet was brought into existence to rise to its full potential. Think about it—have you ever seen a mature six-inch-tall oak tree? We, too, were created to rise to our highest capacity. We were all given special gifts and talents. We were meant to use and develop them. We are not supposed to keep inside that which eagerly desires to be released. We should be using our gifts to create, serve, and be of benefit to humankind and this planet.

It's amazing how much one can learn from a tomato.

Truly believe in yourself.

Cultivate your gifts.

If you want to make positive changes in your life, know that you have the power to do so.

Be thankful for what you have.

Focus on the good in your life.

Be kind and love others.

Go out into the world wearing clean lenses.

Add value to others.

Be consistent.

Learn something new every day.

Don't be afraid to admit that you're wrong.

Seek advice from others.

Take action.

Improve yourself, even a small bit, each day.

Eat natural, healthy foods, including an abundance of colorful fruits and vegetables.

Move your body.

Cherish and take great care of the wonderful gift that has been bestowed upon you.

You are not your genes.

You get to choose.

Small actions will add up over time.

Take baby steps.

Don't rely solely on willpower. Remove temptation.

Understand the power of momentum.

Everything is here to teach us something.

Failure is good, so long as you see the lesson in it.

Be flexible.

Enlarge your perspective.

Expand your comfort zone.

Build good habits.

Expect that life is going to throw you curveballs.

Respond rather than react.

Enjoy life's journey.

Godspeed

AUTHOR'S NOTE

I sincerely enjoyed thinking about and writing this book. I had the opportunity to call to mind many memories as I composed the manuscript. It truly was a labor of love.

It is my hope that you have enjoyed reading this book as much as I have enjoyed writing it. I also genuinely desire that you learned something from my thoughts and experiences that will help you improve your own life, even if only in a small way.

It is my wish that you make good choices each day and enjoy an abundance of health, vitality, happiness, and growth.

Please feel free to reach out to me with any thoughts or questions.

My email is steve@inspiregrowth.life.

All my best,
Steve Piriano, MD

ENDNOTES

1 Miri Potlog Shchory, Lee H. Goldstein, Lidia Arcavi, Renata Shihmanter, Matitiahu Berkovitch, and Amalia Levy, "Increasing Adverse Drug Reaction Reporting—How Can We Do Better?" Plos One, August 13, 2020. https://journals.plos.org/plosone/article?id=10.1371/journal.pone.0235591.

2 Consumer Reports, "Should Children Take Statin Drugs to Lower Their Cholesterol?" last updated June 2010, https://www.consumerreports.org/cro/2012/05/should-children-take-statin-drugs-to-lower-their-cholesterol/index.htm.

3 Centers for Disease Control and Prevention, "High Cholesterol Facts," page last reviewed September 8, 2020, https://www.cdc.gov/cholesterol/facts.htm.

4 Gerald S. Berenson, Sathanur R. Srinivasan, Weihang Bao, William P. Newman, Richard E. Tracy, and Wendy A. Wattigney, "Association between Multiple Cardiovascular Risk Factors and Atherosclerosis in Children and Young Adults," New England Journal of Medicine 338 (1998): 1650–56, https://www.nejm.org/doi/full/10.1056/NEJM199806043382302.

5 Centers for Disease Control and Prevention, "Prevent Type 2 Diabetes in Kids," page last reviewed September 28, 2017, https://www.cdc.gov/diabetes/prevent-type-2/type-2-kids.html.

6 UCLA Health, Ornish Lifestyle Medicine, "The Landmark Lifestyle Heart Trial," accessed January 29, 2021, https://www.uclahealth.org/lifestyle-medicine/workfiles/Lifestyle.pdf.

7 Carra Richling, "Epigenetics: Why Your Lifestyle Choices May Leave Your Family a Legacy of Health," Ornish Living, accessed December 31, 2020, https://www.ornish.com/zine/epigenetics-why-your-lifestyle-choices-may-improve-the-health-of-your-children-and-grandchildren.

8 Katarzyna Szarc vel Szic, Ken Declerck, Melita Vidaković, and Wim Vanden Berghe, "From Inflammaging to Healthy Aging by Dietary Lifestyle Choices: Is Epigenetics the Key to Personalized Nutrition?" Clinical Epigenetics 7 (2015), https://clinicalepigeneticsjournal.biomedcentral.com/articles/10.1186/s13148-015-0068-2.

ALSO BY STEVEN PIRIANO

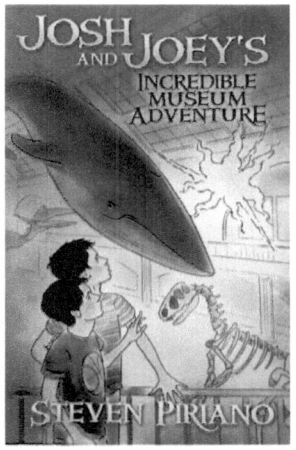

An exciting children's museum quest

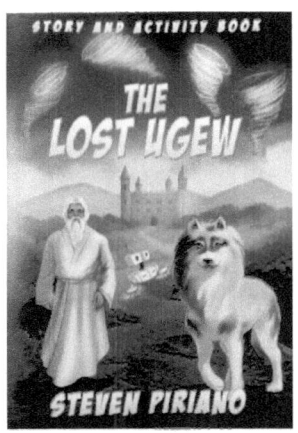

Adventure story and puzzle book

www.ingramcontent.com/pod-product-compliance
Lightning Source LLC
Chambersburg PA
CBHW020535080526
44583CB00013B/864